Overcoming Common Problems

DEPRESSION

Dr Paul Hauck

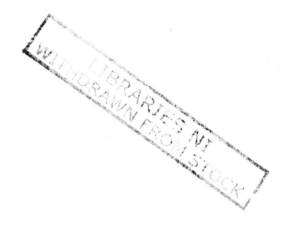

D0237839

sheldon **PRESS**

First published in the USA in 1973 as *Overcoming Depression* by
The Westminster Press, Philadelphia, Pennsylvania

First published in Great Britain in 1974

Sheldon Press
36 Causton Street
London SW1P 4ST

This edition published in 1979

British Library Cataloguing-in-Publication Data
A catalogue record for this book is available
from the British Library.

ISBN 0 85969 168 3

15 17 19 20 18 16

Printed and bound in Great Britain by Biddles Ltd
www.biddles.co.uk

To the most creative thinker I have ever met:

ALBERT ELLIS

ACKNOWLEDGEMENT

Thanks are due to the National Association for Mental Health for permission to quote from *Mind Report No. 12: Psychotherapy: Do We Need More 'Talking Treatment'?*

CONTENTS

PREFACE

Depression is not the most common emotional disturbance. Anger and fear are. However, people do not seek
help for these two afflictions as often as they do for
feelings of guilt, despair, and depression. This is probably
because the latter are recognized as the types of disturbances with which psychotherapists often work, whereas
getting furious or worried is thought to be normal.

Unfortunately, too little has been understood about
depression until now. The poor soul who hated himself,
lived a life feeling inferior, or felt life wasn't worth the
effort, was given the standard medical remedy of anti-
depressant tablets, and sometimes Electro-Convulsive
Therapy (E.C.T.) — all without understanding how he
became depressed.

That time is past. It is now possible, with new methods, for the depressed individual to learn how to get
over his pain, practically forever. Even better news is the
fact that this can often be done in a short time if the
right help and advice is given. This is what I have tried
to show in this book: how people make themselves
depressed, how they keep that depression alive, and how
they can prevent depression in the future.

This book is written for you, the layman, who does
not know the technical psychological terms most books
on this subject use. I have written in an easy-going style
with numerous examples to help explain the points I
am trying to make. Anyone should be able to understand what I have to say, and can most certainly use this
knowledge to fight depression. Some of you will benefit
greatly, I think, even to the point where you can correct

your disturbance almost completely. Others of you will get a good start in overcoming your depressive moods but may need professional help to complete the job.

Even if you are not in need of help yourself, you may have someone dear to you who does. Consider this book a good source of advice for them. You can help your husband or wife, parents, children or friends to overcome depression by telling them what you have learned from studying this book, and how many people have changed their lives after they understood the three main reasons for depression.

If I have accomplished these goals, I will be more than satisfied. So read on! There is hope for you. The material in this book has come from the lives of my patients who were just as depressed as you. They were helped. You will be helped too.

P.A.H.

1

A NEW LOOK AT DEPRESSION

Not long after I graduated, I began work in a community mental health centre. Practically every person who came to me for treatment had uncomfortable mood swings which sometimes went from a low mood back up to normal, or went from a high mood back down to normal. My most baffling patient, however, was the one whose mood hit rock bottom and stayed there.

For a brand-new clinical psychologist this was a most frustrating challenge. The girl I'm referring to was intelligent, well-educated, and came from a secure financial background. She lived in her own home and should have been no more depressed than any number of others whose lives are really not that bad. For these reasons I found it hard to imagine what in the world she was so down about and why she couldn't find a reason to smile.

But Ruth (not her real name) had had a long history of depressions. She was now in her mid-twenties and she had had depressive episodes since early adolescence. She had been in hospital two or three times, as I remember, and she had had courses of tablets of one kind or another and E.C.T.

Ruth was a frequent visitor to the mental health centre, where practically every person on the staff had tried to treat her depression.

I was able to do nothing for her during the first weeks of treatment. If anything, she became rather more depressed, more dependent, and more sure that she'd never come out of this current depressive mood. And she was beginning to convince me that she was right! I listened to her very sympathetically for hours at a time.

I analysed her dreams as I had learned to do according to the teachings of Freud. I took her back into her childhood and attempted to reconstruct her life to see where it had gone sour. In short, I did everything I'd been taught to do, but it wasn't doing her any good. Instead, she wept more when she could see I was becoming unsure of myself. She then began ringing me every morning before I left for the office to tell me she could barely start the day and please couldn't I do or say something that would give her the courage to go on. When she reached the stage where she couldn't sign and address her Christmas cards and her mother had to go over to cook lunch and dinner for Ruth and her children, I felt that it was time to look at my methods very closely and make any changes my common sense suggested.

My psychoanalytic training warned me against working with people other than the patient. That was why I did not follow my natural inclination to encourage Ruth's mother to leave her alone. It was fairly obvious to me that the well-meaning mother was doing so much for the daughter whenever things got a little tough that Ruth never really faced trial and error by herself. Before she could pull herself together when she got low, her mother was there to take over all the responsibilities. Ruth was relieved to have the help, of course, but then she felt inferior because she needed the help and guilty that she accepted it.

At this stage of my professional growth, it never occurred to me to talk Ruth out of feeling guilty for playing the role of a helpless child. Instead, I thought I might make a break in the neurosis by getting the mother to leave her daughter alone. I called Ruth's mother in for a consultation and firmly advised her to visit her daughter not more than once every few days, not to ring her every day, and not to bring over cooked food or to invite Ruth and the children to her home for supper.

Fortunately Ruth's mother accepted my advice and understood fully what I was trying to achieve. It scared her a little to think what would happen to her weak and inadequate daughter if she couldn't rely on someone stronger, but she took my advice literally and stayed away.

Ruth had a very bad time of it for a while but because no one would do things for her she began doing them for herself. I encouraged her to handle her affairs the best she could, not to expect too much of herself, and to consider any little success a positive gain. If she would work at her own speed, I was certain that she could get her confidence back even if it took months. I found myself talking common sense to her rather than keeping quiet as I was psychoanalytically supposed to do. I gave advice until it was coming out of my ears. But she listened, debated over my suggestions, went home and tried some of my advice, and reported to me the following week.

In a matter of a few weeks she was not ringing me every morning, she was coping with her housework and the children, and her mood was definitely lifting. In short, before six months had passed she was out of the woods and her old self again.

I was so curious and pleased by this progress that I decided to write a paper for a forthcoming meeting of local mental health professionals. In the paper I tried to analyse why Ruth had improved and I hazarded the guess that she would probably not have any depressions again if she followed the habits she had been following during the previous months. Looking back on this analysis, I can see how incomplete my understanding was then and how much more quickly Ruth might have improved. I

did not then know how to deal with guilt and self-pity
— her two worst problems — and as a result I dealt with
them only in passing. Happily this was enough, but in
another case it could just as easily not have been.

At the conference I was roundly criticized for suggesting in my paper that I had made a permanent change
in the patient. One of the most respected professionals
there said kind words about how I had brought Ruth
back to full functioning again, but warned me not to
be too optimistic about her chances of staying free from
depression. Everyone knew that depression is largely a
physical problem and that it follows a cycle. Ruth had
lived through a number of cycles already and would
surely go through others.

That was about twenty years ago. Ruth has had only
one serious depressive episode during all those inter-
vening years. She has gone on to college and has been
working and supporting herself nicely all the while. As
proof of her improvement I have received a Christmas
gift each year for the past twenty years from the ex-
depressive who just signs her name 'Ruth'.

A New Theory of Depression

'How can I help you?' is the question I have asked a
great many patients who have come to me for psychological help. More times than I can remember the answer
has been, 'I'm depressed'.

Over the years it became clear to me that depression
was an enormous problem because practically everyone
I had ever treated, or even met socially, had gone through
literally dozens of depressive episodes, most of them
mild, but some of them occasionally quite severe. When
I compare the frequency of depression with other common emotional disturbances, I must conclude that fear

is about as frequent as depression but that anger is the only psychological condition more frequent. I will touch on anger in this book because some rather good material has been published on the subject lately. But depression is still in a no-man's-land; the condition has been written about at some length, to be sure, but not in a way that offers the average reader much help.

I am writing this book to pass on to others some of the newest thinking about neurosis, and to offer them a new theory of depression which I have formulated and tested in well over a hundred cases.

Best of all, I find that applying this theory of depression to my own moods can get me over episodes that would ordinarily have put me in a nose-dive to misery. Before I practised this new thinking I had as many problems with the miseries as anyone. Being rejected made me feel inferior and guilty and I would have to stay by myself for hours or days before I came out of it. If I did a job badly or did poorly in exams, it really worried me and I would have to fight my way out. Again, it would take hours or days. And when I was treated unfairly my self-pity really welled up.

Thank God that was long ago. I have had many things happen to me in my life and not all of them have been pleasant. But I admit I have been lucky enough to be happily married, to have three lovely daughters, and to have parents in good health. Nor have I been unemployed since leaving university. So perhaps I have not had the same reasons to be seriously depressed that others have. I'm sure I'd have reacted badly to a misfortune in any of those personal areas of my life. In fact, any of the usual misfortunes would still jolt me today, but I am also sure I would cope with them so much better now that I have learned about depression and how to handle it. As a result, I have not been depressed for so many years I cannot honestly count them. I can ride the bad times (provided they are not overwhelming) and I have taught hundreds of others to do the same. And this is the important point. It is not the catastrophies one must learn to handle as much as the small daily trials. If we can deal with everyday disappointments, failures, or rejections, we have practically got the better of the depression problem. It was once thought that depression was something your parents passed down to you, like your brown hair and blue eyes. That's why so little was done about this condition for so long. People gave up hope of trying to change something supposedly given them by heredity. But, as opinion began to change, doctors tried medicine and E.C.T. and both worked up to a point, especially with the more severe depressions. Milder depression, however, the sort you would talk over with your husband, wife, or best friend, never received much professional attention and so failed to be studied and explained. True, Freud saw the obvious connection between guilt and depression, but he then got on the wrong track by insisting that the guilt was caused when a child gets sexy fantasies about his parents. Some of his other ideas made some sense, but again they weren't much help to the man in the street who'd just got the sack.

It may well be that we are all born with a tendency towards depression: some of us have more, some less, than others. This, however, can't be the sole cause of feeling blue. If it was, there'd be little that anyone could do. Instead we are able to teach people how to get over depression and so it would only seem reasonable to suppose that someone else taught them to be depressed in the first place. When you get upset in any way, you are doing what comes fairly naturally, because you inherited an imperfect head and you were taught and well trained to be irrational by a whole collection of people who also inherited imperfect heads. Practically everywhere you look, in magazines, in films, or on TV, and no matter to whom you listen, whether it be your parents, teachers, or friends, you are being trained to be neurotic by these forces and don't know it. They have taught you to be a first-class depressive and it's now up to you to undo the damage they unwittingly did to you.

You must learn new ways to think, create new attitudes to people and events. How can you do it? By considering depression as a subject to study just like geometry, history, or art. Consider a psychiatrist's advice to be a course in healthy living, given by a teacher who assigns you reading, asks you to come to a classroom-office once a week or less, and conducts his class for one pupil usually but sometimes a group of students.

What I'm really getting at is that you don't need to feel there is something different or weird about yourself because you have the blues. You are the way you are mainly because you were trained to be that way in exactly the same way you learned to speak the language of your parents. What you learned was mostly rubbish, but you learned it well. If you can do that, then it shouldn't be too hard to learn some sensible ideas for a change. You have proved that you are able to grasp neurotic ideas. What is to prevent you from grasping healthy ideas? It won't be as easy as it sounds, but it can be done.

Yes, a book can actually rid some of you of your depressive habits. It can show you what you are doing wrong, and teach you which of your thinking habits are hurting you and which habits you should replace them with.

It would be unrealistic to suggest that every kind of depression can be eliminated by reading a book, because depression can come in various degrees of severity. One can feel vaguely low because an expected phone call doesn't come; then again, one can feel so guilty over a car accident that a spell in hospital and E.C.T. are needed. This book will help those with the milder problems the most. But it can help the more depressed as well. Even if a severe problem is only made less severe, instead of being totally conquered, wouldn't it be worth the effort of learning how we became depressed and how to go about reducing the condition?

Some depressions are caused by physical factors, not by psychological ones. The former should be dealt with by your family doctor. Some depressions, especially when you seem to get depressed for no apparent reason, may result from changes in the level of biogenic amines in the brain and disturbances of water and electrolytes balance or from a condition called hypoglycemia. This means that the blood has very little glucose, the food required by every cell in the body. Hypoglycemics feel restless, dizzy, irritable, or depressed, or all of these. Some authorities think that persons who have certain forms of mental retardation and schizophrenia, and most alcoholics, are all suffering from low blood sugar.

If you suspect that you fall into the category of the hypoglycemic, see your doctor and ask for a test. If, however, you can point to something in your life that you believe started the depression, then you probably have a case of psychological depression and should read on.

Three Causes of Depression

1. Self-blame

If you are constantly criticizing yourself, hating yourself, thinking that you are the worst human being alive, you will most certainly become depressed. It makes practically no difference what you blame yourself for, just so long as you give yourself hell for it. It might be because you didn't get promotion, or because you didn't win the annual darts championship, or even because someone forgot to say 'Hello' to you. Just blame yourself and you have a depression coming on. And if you blame yourself enough, you will become quite disturbed, probably feel like crying, become silent and moody, and you may even want to jump into the nearest river.

If you blame yourself only a little, you will just feel uncomfortable and certainly moody. This condition is not a serious one, but it could spoil an evening's entertainment, ruin a party or a visit, and make those around you feel glum.

2. Self-pity

The second way to get depressed is to feel sorry for yourself. Cry into your beer when you're not treated fairly and you will soon be depressed. Put on a long face just to get sympathy and you're on your way to a depression. Think that the world owes you a living and when you find out how unfair life can be, you're depressed.

This will come as a real surprise to millions of people, but they had better learn it's neurotic to insist that others treat us fairly, that our kindnesses be returned with kindness, and that the world has to be a decent place. If we believe this nonsense, we are bound to become depressed and to feel hurt and angry when things don't go the way we think they should.

If you want to avoid depression, you are going to have to learn that unfair and unkind behaviour in exchange for your loving efforts is the rule rather than the exception. The sooner you realize the world will always be that way, the healthier a person you will become.

3. Other Pity

Just as you can get depressed if you break your own leg, you can become depressed if someone else breaks his. Because there is endless suffering in the world, there is endless opportunity to identify with the troubles of millions of poor souls, to say nothing of those in one's immediate family. And indeed, their troubles and heartaches are real and sometimes pathetic. But if you pity the child with crutches, the man whose house burnt down, the mother whose son died in the war, you will become just as depressed as if you blamed yourself or pitied yourself. The depression will look the same, and can reach the same depths of misery, regardless of what's provoking it. The only thing you can be sure of is that you're in pain of the worst sort.

There you have it, the three reasons why, in my view, people become emotionally depressed. In the following pages you can learn why you blame yourself and think you are right to do so; why you pity yourself and feel correct and justified in doing so; and why you pity others and feel squeamish about doing otherwise. Furthermore, you can also learn why you are wrong, foolish, and totally mistaken to hate yourself under *any* conditions; why pitying yourself only makes you your own worst enemy; and why pitying others undermines their self-confidence. I will explain to you how you justify these actions and how you must change your beliefs to avoid future depressions. So read on, all you who are depressed. You have nothing to lose but much to gain.

2

SELF-BLAME

When I tell my patients they would be much better off never to feel guilt, they look at me as though I had lost my senses. 'How is it possible never to feel guilt when it's impossible to behave perfectly?' they ask. The answer is really quite simple: admit that you *are* guilty when you have done something you think was wrong, immoral, or needlessly painful to others. Do that and nothing more. I assure you that you'll be so undisturbed by your objectionable behaviour that you will begin to look at your actions in a calm and objective way. You will even think over your actions so that you can probably avoid doing the same again in the future.

What most people do, however, is admit that they *are* guilty of wrong behaviour and then they *feel* guilty over that behaviour. It is that second step which causes the trouble. It convinces them that they are terrible, evil, and worthless people because they behaved badly.

And what does it mean to feel guilt? It means you have *labelled* yourself by your behaviour. The process usually goes something like this: 'I am guilty of being rude to that waiter. That means I'm bad.' 'I'm guilty of belittling my wife. I'm worthless.'

You have been *judging yourself by your behaviour*. If you behave well, you think you're marvellous. If you behave badly, you think you're worthless. But should you? Must we rate ourselves? Must we pin a medal on our chests for being kind to an old lady crossing the street and must we hate ourselves if we push an old lady into the street?

You're immediately going to tell me that we *should*

feel guilty for behaving badly. You're going to insist there has to be something terribly wrong with anyone who would hurt an old lady, shout at an innocent waiter, or run down his wife in public. Such a person just must be worthless, wicked, evil and just plain bad. Not so. There's always a good reason why you may have behaved badly; a reason so good, in fact, that you have every right to forgive yourself.

Three Reasons for Not Blaming Yourself

1. Stupidity

By stupidity I mean not having the intelligence to do as well as you'd like to do. If a person is mentally retarded, we can hardly expect him to behave in a faultless way. And even if he were not intellectually retarded, he could still be so limited in his intelligence in specialized ways that we could easily forgive him for doing badly. Let's take the example of the retarded child first.

Johnny has an I.Q. of about 60. He is about eight years old and loves to pick up things and finger them. One day he comes into your home, finds a box of matches and plays with them. Accidentally he sets the room on fire and someone gets hurt. What he has done is a most unfortunate thing, but would we say Johnny is a bad and evil child? I hope not. It was, after all, not his wickedness that drove him to play with the matches, it was a child's curiosity. His low intelligence prevented him from sensing the danger he was in. Even if he had burned down the whole house and killed everyone in it, the facts would remain unchanged. Johnny would *be* guilty of a terrible act but would be foolish to *feel* guilty over it since he was behaving in the only way retarded children can act with matches: unintelligently. It would also be foolish for the adults concerned to scold and shout at the boy and to try to make him depressed. In short we would judge the act without also judging the child. His actions were wicked, he was not.

Suppose we now take a more usual example, this time a young girl. Her parents want her to play the piano. It seems, however, that she has very little talent for the instrument—or for music, for that matter. So she inevitably does poorly, learns slowly, and has no feel for the music. In a word, she is unintelligent where music is concerned. It is as though, in this one area of her life, she is retarded and incapable of ever doing well.

Would you think the girl was wicked merely because she played the piano badly? I would certainly hope not. The temptation to rate the girl by her inferior piano-playing usually doesn't occur to us, because nothing really dreadful has happened.

2. Ignorance

Suppose a person is not retarded and does something really wicked. Should we then conclude that that person is worthless and evil?

Imagine you are a young father and your wife took the evening off and left you to care for your new baby. The child cries and you find that his nappy needs changing. One of the big safety pins gets jammed, so you carelessly push too forcefully to open it and injure the baby.

Again, it makes sense to say that you *are* guilty of hurting the baby, but surely you would agree that you don't need to *feel* guilty. You wouldn't, of course, feel glad over the mistake. That would be highly neurotic to say the least.

Feeling guilty, however, would mean that you think you *should not* have hurt the baby, and that is foolish. You are, after all, a clumsy, inexperienced father who loves his child and wants to make him comfortable. In the circumstances it would be rather surprising if you did not hurt the child from time to time until you gained more skill. Your problem is not that you are a hateful person for hurting the baby, but that you are ignorant. More practice will give you more skill in baby matters.

Ignorance means that you have not yet learned a skill, whereas stupidity means that you can never learn it no matter how much practice you get. Even a genius can be ignorant and not do a great many things well until he has had the opportunity to learn them.

Mothers often have a big problem with guilt feelings about the poor job they have done in bringing up their children. Perhaps the children have taken to drugs, become pregnant, or dropped out of school. When such instances are studied carefully it is easy to find numerous examples of poor child-rearing practices. In fact, I often tell these mothers that I agree with them, that they are awful mothers and have brought their children up badly, but I immediately stress the fact that they have no legitimate right to hate themselves for their many blunders. Whatever they did in bringing up their children they did with the best of intentions and love. They may have loved too much, or been too eager to protect their children from making serious mistakes and nagged them over-conscientiously.

Their problem was not that they are worthless people, just poor mothers. And why shouldn't they be? Many of them had emotional problems of their own. Most, however, did not have the right information on how to handle many of the problems of child-rearing. If they were ignorant about how to deal with a rebellious youngster, should they scold themselves and *feel* guilty because they *are* guilty?

I take a very different attitude about such mistakes. I

point out to these women that most of them have never had a course in psychology. Many of them have not read the best books on child-rearing. I urge them not to be too hard on themselves or feel guilty over the faulty rearing of their children, because they could not do what they were not taught. Most of them were merely following the faulty techniques practiced on them by their own well-meaning parents. And why shouldn't they? Why shouldn't the child-rearing methods they saw all their lives being practiced on them, be imitated?

Again, it is their ignorance, their lack of knowledge of better methods, which created their problems with the children, not some rotten quality within them that they should blame themselves for.

Now let's look at a really serious case. Suppose a teenager is learning to drive. He comes to a road crossing at lunchtime just as a group of children are crossing. Instead of stepping on the brake pedal, he accidentally steps on the accelerator, goes onto the crossing, and kills several of the children.

It goes without saying that the parents of these children would be very much disturbed by this tragedy and would want to lynch the boy. His parents might also be furious with him. Worst of all, the boy himself would be inclined to blame himself so severely that he would almost certainly become depressed. He *was* the guilty party who killed the children. Shouldn't he *feel* guilty too?

No! He should not feel guilty, because he has an excellent reason for having the accident: he is inexperienced, untrained, and still very awkward behind the wheel of a car. If he had had more practice, he would most certainly not have made such a blunder. Again, he is guilty because he was ignorant, not evil.

You may have the feeling in your heart that something

is wrong, even dangerous with this way of thinking. If we don't blame people for their serious mistakes, if we don't want them to feel guilty over someone's death, then what is to stop people from doing wrong all the time and not even minding it either?

You have forgotten that stupid and ignorant people did not want to behave badly in the first place, or that they did not realize that their behaviour was wrong even while engaged in it (as with the retarded population). In any event, you are of course quite correct that something must be done about retarded boys who could walk into your house and accidentally set it on fire. And we must certainly do something about the young driver so that he does not get so confused when coming to a crossing that he cannot tell which pedal is the brake and which is the accelerator.

In the first case we will try to be more careful about leaving our doors unattended so that the local children cannot wander in at any time. We can also see to it that we keep matches out of the reach of children, and do the same with guns, knives, and other dangerous objects.

For young people taking driving lessons, we could perhaps give them more exercises for reacting quickly to the brake, and do this in the safety of the driving school grounds, on an isolated road, or in a field, before letting them drive in city streets. That is what we should do about preventing these kinds of accidents. Screaming at the person after the damage is done does pitifully little good and may do a great deal of harm. We confuse him with so much guilt feeling that he often does not stop to think about how the accident happened in the first place and what he should do to avoid it again in the future.

3. Disturbance

By now the thought will have occurred to you that there

is one class of behaviours that are unforgivable: those which are committed deliberately with full knowledge of what the consequences will be. Take the case of a bright student at university who has an I.Q. of about 130 but who is wasting his time so much he is about to be sent down. He knows he's in danger of being thrown out. He knows that by doing his work and giving up girls and drink he could pass his course easily. So you're inclined to insist he should feel guilty because he's intelligent and knows what is happening to his career. Still he stupidly heads straight for disaster.

Apparently we cannot excuse his behaviour on the grounds that he is stupid (retarded) or ignorant. We can, however, excuse it on the grounds that he would have to be disturbed. How else are we going to understand such foolish behaviour? In other words, such a person is not evil or worthless because he is wasting his parents' money and sadly disappointing them. Such a person is neurotic, vengeful, or afraid. Such a person has emotional problems which make him act as though he were an idiot. And if you had his emotional troubles, you'd probably act the same way.

I have known a number of promising students who behaved exactly as I described in the example. When their problems were analysed they always boiled down to the person being so afraid he would not live up to the godlike expectations of his parents that he just couldn't face the defeat he knew he would experience if he really tried. When you have been told all your life that you're marvellous and intelligent, and are sure to become the chairman of a bank, you have a heavy burden to live up to. Rather than let your family know that you might just be an ordinary person, you let yourself fail because you can always blame the failure on your not trying, rather than on a limited ability which they always insisted you did not have. Then you can even feel less guilt by saying you failed at university because you played around, rather than because you weren't a genius after all.

Now suppose it isn't fear at all. Then it might be spite, another serious emotional problem. In this case your parents forced you to study medicine, but you really hate it. By fooling around you get back at them for not letting you become an artist, even if it hurts you also. Your results are suffering all round — including the qualifications you'll need if you are ever to go to art school. You are also developing some powerfully bad habits that you'll have to overcome if and when you can get your parents to change their minds. You know all this, but you can't do a thing about it. You are neurotic, and all the reasoning in the world will not change your behaviour for the time being. Your goal in life is either to avoid looking inadequate, since you think that you are worthless unless you are a top student, or to be so angry with your parents that nothing else matters.

Never Blame Yourself for Anything, At Any Time, Anywhere

When you *feel* guilty because you *are* guilty over some misdeed, you are blaming yourself. That is one of the most unhealthy acts you can perform. It is one I want to teach you never to commit and in the following pages I hope to show you why you are neurotic if you blame yourself, what self-blame leads to, and how to fight it. First, let me explain for a moment exactly what I mean by blame.

Blame involves a double attack: one against your actions, the other against yourself as a person. If you spill ink on the furniture, you are only sensible to call yourself clumsy. You are not sensible, however, to attack yourself and call yourself all sorts of ugly names because you may be clumsy. You may be careless. You may be unco-ordinated. You may even do it because you are spiteful. But you are not an outcast because of any of these reasons. If you think you are, then you have already blamed yourself.

I know of a man who accidentally killed a pedestrian in a car accident. Naturally he strongly disapproved of his careless driving, but he decided that because he had been the unwitting cause of another man's death he should never forgive himself. That is blame. He blamed himself for years. He was depressed on and off, to a greater or lesser degree, for about ten years of his life before he learned that his depression and self-blame were quite neurotic.

Self-blame is like giving yourself a school report. At school it is fairly accurate to say that you got 'A' for geography or history, 'B' for English, etc. That doesn't make *you* an 'A' or a 'B' person, though. You must separate the subject from yourself as a human being. If you do not do this, you will believe that you are fine when you receive 'A's' and worthless when you receive 'F's'. This is precisely what is often done. And the same applies to non-school subjects. It applies to everyday behaviour. A woman who goes against her religious teachings and has an abortion may very likely have performed an immoral act in her eyes, but she also becomes an *immoral human being* in her own eyes. She rates her*self* by her actions. That means that the only times she will be a worthwhile person is when she behaves perfectly and above fault. It is obvious that people who follow this philosophy are doomed to be depressed a good deal of the time, for how often can any of us ever behave in a faultless manner? At this point, my patients usually raise this question: 'How can I separate my behaviour from myself? My actions are me.' In the following chapter I will go into the techniques of overcoming depression and learning to separate one's behaviour from oneself. For the present I want first to convince you of the utter danger of self-blame by showing all the unfortunate consequences that result from it.

Blame Is a Violent Act Against Yourself

Stop for a moment and think what you do to yourself when you blame yourself. First you think of yourself as unworthy of belonging to the human race. You see yourself as a species apart from all others. You smear yourself with verbal filth so that you stink to yourself even if others cannot smell you. You tar and feather yourself with invisible hate and loathing. Sometimes you physically punish yourself with burning cigarettes or you cut yourself with razor blades. And always you treat yourself as though others should spit on you and avoid you like the plague. Now that is violence, wouldn't you agree?

Suppose now that someone else were to do all these acts to you. Wouldn't you fight for your very life not to be treated in such a shameful way? Of course you would. You would have to be crazy not to. But do you stop this violence when it is *you* who is doing it? Not at all. You relish it. You think you have it coming to you. It even feels good to you because you believe that through all of this self-torture you are cleansing yourself of all your sins.

If it is so good to suffer when *you* do it, why is it wrong if someone else does it? In fact, if you want to be sensible and realistic about it, all you self-blamers should go to jail and really get a dose of punishment, or volunteer for suicide squads, or work in leper colonies. Strange as it seems, this is precisely what some consistent self-blamers actually do. They expose themselves to danger, bankruptcy, failure, all in the belief that they have it coming to them because they're worthless. Most self-blamers, however, don't go this far. They punish themselves in private, curse their existence to themselves while trying to hide their self-hatred from others, and do not ever see that they are being monstrously unfair to themselves.

Blame Is Always Dangerous

Not only is blame wrong when directed at you, by yourself; it is wrong and dangerous when directed at others. In the latter case it generates hatred, anger, and violence. If you remember what I've just pointed out about blame against oneself, you will easily see why blame against others does the same. When others behave badly you are naturally inclined to rate them as wicked also. They become the same as their deeds. Good deeds, and you think you are dealing with good humans; bad deeds and you're dealing with bad people. Rubbish! Again we confuse the person with his actions.

Practically all the violence, war, torture, and murder in the world can be traced to this awful belief that (a) there are bad people in the world and (b) bad people should be severely blamed and punished for their evil acts. Certainly they should be locked up for our safety, but to kill or punish them is doing no more than they did to come to our attention.

Let's not go to extremes. Most of us don't even know a murderer, so a look at an everyday event would help explain the dangers of blame a great deal better. Your husband has just bought a car and didn't consult you about it. You didn't even want another car, but you are willing to overlook that. However, you didn't even have a chance to select the model or the colour. And after all you've done for him! You have been more than fair with him. You don't spend five pence without first consulting him. Now you decide that this is terribly unfair (and you're absolutely correct), so you hit him with everything that has ever annoyed you about him. When you have given him a good tongue-lashing, you throw something, and for the finale you try to make him feel utterly wretched by going to your bedroom and weeping. If you have a bathroom with a lock on it, that is even better.

This is not a fairy tale. This is an event that takes place every so often in practically every household. In some homes it's as daily a ritual as washing up.

The wife in the above example has blamed her husband for being thoughtless. In effect she says to herself: 'He *behaved* wrongly. *He* is bad.' And ninety-nine percent of the world would agree with her. But I protest. How is she wrong? For one thing, her husband is a human being, made imperfectly just as she was. That means he must have some faults. If she doesn't want thoughtlessness as one of his big faults, then what would she be satisfied with? Would she be happier if he were a rapist? or a child molester? or an embezzler? No? Then perhaps she ought to accept him with this fault and go about calmly trying to break him of this habit, instead of giving him reason to hate her so much he just might go out and buy an elephant without consulting her.

This kind of blame is dangerous because it drives people away, breaks up marriages, helps create guilt and depression in the victim, and plays hell with your blood pressure and ulcers. One cannot be furious at another without paying a price. I have known some people who were told by their doctors that they had bad hearts and should not get upset for any reason. Yet these same people go on, day after day, getting angry about a million things and *they* have to pay the price for it. Someone once said that anger was the price *you* paid for another person's mistakes.

Self-blamers Are Conceited

When you think back over the times when you felt very guilty you can probably remember only how inferior you felt, how untouchable you must have seemed to others, and how totally unworthy you had become. Depressed people can usually be described as humble, lacking self-confidence, and having a very low opinion of themselves. To suggest that these self-loathers are fundamentally conceited sounds preposterous. Yet such is clearly the case.

An adolescent girl recently told me that she had become pregnant and felt like killing herself. She went on to say she felt dirty and ashamed. For all the world her behaviour could be described as anything but conceit. That is why it almost knocked her out of the chair when I suggested that she was one of the most conceited persons I had ever met.

'Me? Conceited?' she asked in amazement.

'Yes, you. You think you're so unbelievably good that you shouldn't make mistakes or blunder in any way at all.'

'But that's true. I shouldn't have become pregnant, I knew better, but I let it happen anyway.'

'What if one of your girl friends had become pregnant? Would you blame her? Would you want to kill her? Would you refuse to speak to her? Would you shun her company just as you think others should shun you? Like hell you would! Unless you're very different from most people, you'd go up to your girl friend, put your arm around her, and give her all the support and love you could show. And you'd mean it too.'

'Yes,' she said, 'I'm sure I would. But isn't that different?'

'I suppose it is,' I answered. 'People like her are expected to get pregnant. But superhuman people like yourself, well, that's different. *You* aren't supposed to make mistakes. *You* can't be impulsive and romantic. That's what one expects from the common herd, like your girl friend. But *you*, ah, that's different. I suppose you must belong to a different species of mankind.'

It gradually dawned on the girl that she *was* being high-handed when she could not forgive herself for a careless act, whereas she wouldn't hesitate to do the same for her friend.

This is an underlying trait of all self-blamers. They cannot stand the ugly fact that they are just human, faulty, mistake makers. No amount of work will ever change that trait completely. Still they go on endlessly, neurotically demanding that their behaviour has to be better than others' and that unless they stop their wrong-doings immediately, they deserve the worst kind of treatment.

It is high time we fully appreciated what it means to be human.

Suppose you were God and you decided to populate your planets with perfect creatures. You could make them all wise, with supercolossal intelligence, amazingly quick reflexes, and completely without periods of youth or old age. After all, even God cannot make a perfect baby, because by definition a baby is an undeveloped and ignorant creature. And God would want to eliminate the aged, for how else could he have a world full of error-free people if he allowed them to grow old and senile and thereby lose the alertness that made these people so perfect? He would, therefore, have to create people who are born with young bodies and middle-aged minds, and that is the way they would be forever, or until they died (assuming that God wanted them to live for only a specified period). There would be no ageing process as we know it, for that would surely introduce faulty behaviour. Therefore, in a universe of perfect beings it would have to be 'Here today, gone tomorrow'.

On the other hand, if you were God, you could decide to make the creatures who will inherit your universe imperfect. But if you did that, your expectations of these poor mortals ought certainly to be quite different from the expectations of a planet full of perfect beings. From mortals we should expect a long period of learning, as long as sixteen or eighteen years before these creatures could even consider being on their own. And as these mortals got older we would expect them to lose their quickness, their intellectual sharpness, and to deteriorate slowly in all respects. But even during their best years we would expect these normal human beings to do all manner of silly and stupid things. In other words, we would expect some of these people to commit murder, suicide, theft, and all manner of atrocities. Mothers from this group will beat their babies to death. Fathers from this group will declare wars for their sons to die in. These people will hate very easily as well as love very easily. Though they will be capable of remarkable achievements, such as the conquest of diseases, and the exploration of outer space, these same people will mess things up by polluting their air, saving so many people that their planet threatens to become overpopulated, and building so many atomic bombs that their entire world could be blown apart.

All of this sounds perfectly reasonable to me because I really do accept the fact that man is man, that man is imperfect, and that he cannot help being a fool a great deal of the time.

Nevertheless, there are millions of people who will still go on saying that man should not be violent, that one's children should not die, and that accidents should not happen. How stupid can we be?

How much better it would be to say: 'It would be *better* if we were not so violent. How much *nicer* existence would be if our loved ones did not die. And wouldn't it be *wonderful* if we did not have accidents?' These statements make sense because they express wishes and preferences, not demands or necessities. Demanding something merely because you want something is certain to lead to disturbance if you don't get your way. Stop demanding perfect behaviour from yourself, and accept your actions for the unavoidable conditions they are, and you are sure to be more self-loving as well as more loving towards other people. Give up your conceit. Remember: God chose to make people according to the second plan I outlined, not the first.

Self-blamers Are Cowards

Guilt is a fantastically successful method of keeping people from committing certain acts. Murder is less frequent than it is, not only because one gets a stiff jail sentence for it but because we would dread living with our guilty conscience afterwards. People all over the world have behaved in a law-abiding way because their sense of guilt would hurt them too much to do otherwise. There's no denying the efficiency of making our consciences the guardians over our conduct.

Unfortunately the price we pay for using guilt in this way is enormous, for not only does it prevent us from behaving badly, it very frequently prevents us from behaving courageously and sensibly. When Shakespeare pointed out that conscience makes cowards of us all, he was expressing this very idea. I would like to show you how a guilty conscience can make such a weakling out of you that you end up allowing others to take the most unkind advantage of you, and how it can make you deny your own interests to the point where you wonder if you have a mind of your own, or if your life belongs to you.

Bill was a particularly good example of what happens to a person who feels guilty. Once during his marriage he had an affair, but his wife never found out about it. Afraid she would reject him, Bill kept the secret to himself for over ten years. During this time he felt that he had no right to assert himself against his wife's unreasonable behaviour, and she, sensing that he would never fight for his own rights, tended to take ever greater advantage of him. It got so bad between them that he hated her for her unreasonableness, and hated himself for being a coward and not kicking her in the teeth. And she hated him because he never showed any gumption and let her figuratively wipe her feet on him.

Spending some time alone with him, I learned about his affair and how he justified his weakness and fear. He could see quite easily that he had been very cowardly over the years, but he could not understand at all when I insisted he had no need to feel guilty about the affair, and that the sooner he confessed to his wife, the sooner she could not hold that invisible guilt over his head.

I tried to help Bill accept himself and stop blaming himself. When he at last realised that his affair resulted from his low self-esteem, which is a psychological problem and not some wicked character trait, he was able to confess his indiscretions to his wife. As predicted, their relationship changed a great deal after she got over the initial shock.

'When I realize what I've put up with all these years,' Bill later said, 'I could really kick myself. Just because

I did one thing I was ashamed of, I let that woman have her way, let her say things to me, make all kinds of demands, and I felt I just had to take it. It never occurred to me to ask what the hell she was doing to *me*. If I'd treated her the way she treated me, what with all her selfishness, I would have had plenty to blame myself for. But do you think she gave a moment's thought to the way she was treating me?'

Bill's new-found assertiveness gave him an added bonus: his wife gained new respect for him. As she put it: 'Of course I think more of Bill now. Why, to compare his strength now with the feeble character I was married to before makes me think perhaps I was hoping to make him so sick of my nagging that he would finally get some guts and act like a man.'

One of the most interesting and unusual consequences of a guilty conscience was observed in a teenage girl who was not only depressed but heard voices telling her to kill her mother or to kill herself. Mother and daughter argued a good deal, and there were the usual scenes and ugly words when things got very nasty. Though the mother meant well and wanted only to correct her daughter, she failed to see how hostile the girl was becoming at being told how to run her life all day. It took a few years of this warfare before the hatred got so intense that the girl did not even want to recognize it. That is when she developed the auditory hallucinations.

Sometimes the girl could ignore the voices, but often they bothered her during a normal conversation when talking to a friend or making a purchase, for example. This really unnerved her because she couldn't carry on two conversations at once and she couldn't let the person with her know she was troubled by inner 'voices'.

The first time I learned about this symptom was during a group therapy session. I asked the other members of the group for their ideas about what the girl should do to stop the voices. Their thoughts ran along the following line: find an excuse to leave the scene; talk more loudly to drown out the murderous suggestions; begin laughing to convince herself the whole thing was ridiculous; and finally, say nothing until the voices ceased. I explained why none of these solutions would probably work and then told them what I thought would do the trick. A female member of the group almost fainted when I suggested, 'We've got to convince her not to feel guilty for wanting to kill her mother.'

Let me explain my thinking this way: the more you worry about a thing happening, the more likely it is to happen. The young lady was always very conscious of these threatening voices and she was quite alarmed by them as well. They never would have got out of control had she not made an earthshaking event out of having the feelings of murder in the first place. Had she taken them calmly, she could have laughed them off easily enough. To this end, I advised her to consider her anger fairly normal, to realize that she had had these feelings a number of times—probably hundreds—and still had never acted on them, and to forgive her mother for frustrating her since her mother too was only human and trying her best to help her daughter. Each time the voices plagued her she was to react as calmly as possible, do nothing about suppressing them, feel no guilt, and in time they would certainly diminish in importance.

Inside one month the voices had gone almost completely. If they returned sporadically, she analysed her angry feelings and talked herself out of them. And because no one in the group thought she was a terrible person for hating her mother, she lost her sense of panic over them. It was only then that she confronted her mother in a healthy way and didn't allow herself to be dominated. This action prevents the numerous frustrations that normally set her off.

The last example of guilt making cowards of us is that of John. He was an alcoholic who frequently got drunk because his father wanted someone to drink with and to make the rounds of the bars with. John was now in AA and trying his best to stay dry, but every once in a while he would come to me depressed because he had refused to drink with dear old father, and on one recent occasion he refused to let his father take his three children with him on his tour of the bars. At such times, the father would appeal directly to John's sense of guilt and point out all that he had done for John over the years, and how it was John's duty as a son to grant his father these simple favours. John held firm and refused, but it tore him up inside to do so.

I attempted to show John that his father was being nothing more than an emotional baby by demanding these ridiculous things and that it would hardly kill the old boy to be refused. Then I showed John how he could very easily deny his father a great number of favours without feeling guilty if he could decide in his own mind that the issues were important.

'John, if your father told you he had a strong hankering to burn your house down just so he could have some excitement, you surely wouldn't let him go ahead and do it, would you?'

'Of course not.'

'Or suppose your father wanted to use your living room for a toilet, would you let him?'

'Of course not.'

'But, John, suppose he told you how a son is supposed to please his father, how you owe him for years of devotion, how he thinks you are ungrateful, inconsiderate, and so on because you won't let him burn down your house or use your rug as a place to relieve himself. Would any of that make any difference?'

'I know what you're getting at, doctor, but that's different.'

'Different? What's so different about those examples and what the old boy has actually done to you already? He's helped make you an alcoholic and practically ruined your marriage, and now he's suggesting he put your girls in danger just so he can have some company. No, John, I can't go along with your reasoning. If you can refuse him some items, you can refuse him two more which are immensely important to you.'

And he did see the point. Rather than let his father play on his guilt, John became firm with the old man, accepted the temporary rejection that followed, and did himself and his children a world of good. None of this would have been possible, however, if he had not conquered his guilt.

Feeling Guilty Makes Your Behaviour Worse

It is drummed into us that it's moral to feel guilty over misdeeds, on the grounds that the pain connected with the guilt will prove so unpleasant we won't commit the same fault again. If this is what actually happened, I'd be the first to suggest we develop all the guilt we can and so become less and less error prone. Unfortunately this is not the case. In fact, the *opposite* behaviour works better, i.e., don't blame yourself *at all*, but analyse your errors and sins, and then try hard not to repeat them. Blaming yourself for your sins convinces you that better behaviour is all but impossible, and that worse behaviour is exactly what a beast like you needs for punishment. Besides, how else can you impress your error on your memory if you don't bleed inside because of it?

Take the case of Lucy. She married, her husband left for service overseas, she was lonely and had an affair. Although she had moral pangs about this romance, she enjoyed it enough to block out any thought of stopping it, or of blaming herself severely. But it ended in six months and she then found herself in the arms of another man almost immediately. Now she began to hate herself. It was at this point she decided she must be a whore, a depraved human being who was above help, and who might just as well go out and lay any male who took a liking to her. One night after attending a party, she noticed that one of the men at the party was following her in his car. What did she do? The only consistent thing a 'whore' could do. She stopped her car, walked back to his, and made love. Then she went home. I received a call that evening from a very weepy girl, contemplating suicide, and asking for help.

It didn't take long to get her to see what she was doing to herself. She changed completely when she realized that self-blame had convinced her she was all bad, instead of just foolish and unfaithful. I never once agreed with her that her actions were harmless. The way she was jumping around from bed to bed was serious, could give her a disease or make her pregnant, and was terribly unfair to her husband. But I insisted that she did those reckless things because she was so disturbed due to her guilt that she had no choice but to continue her self-punishing tactics. When she understood this, the problem was neatly nipped in the bud.

It will not hurt you much to blame yourself just a little. It is the severe and constant self-blame you must watch out for. When you believe you are unworthy, you will see to it that nothing worthy happens to you. The worst enemies we have are ourselves. The boy who is told that he will never amount to anything because he has cheated in a test, and that he should be ashamed of all the pain he has caused his mother—that boy is sure to feel unworthy of his mother's love, and he will do whatever it takes to get his mother to detest him. After all, his mother has told him repeatedly he is not worthy of her love, and can his mother be wrong?

Self-acceptance is the medicine to cure this illness—acceptance of one's weaknesses, one's human faults and habits, while all the time trying hard to overcome these annoying human frailties we all inherit when we are born. Forgiveness for others, but also forgiveness for ourselves is the great lesson the self-blamer must learn.

Religion and Self-blame

To some of you the points I've made about never blaming yourself sound wicked and sinful. You might conclude that I advocate all kinds of immoral acts, all sorts of violence, and that I encourage people to do these things without even feeling guilty about them. This is certainly not true. In fact, I maintain that (a) most people who think they are religious are not, (b) most people who thing they are leading a good life as outlined in the Bible are often doing just the opposite, and (c) what I have said about never blaming yourself is very Christian and (d) is supported by the Bible.

Our religions want us to be happy people, content with ourselves and loving toward others. When we err, we are told by our faiths that it is human to do so. We should forgive ourselves. We should forgive those who trespass against us also. Remember? When you do not blame others for their errors, you are forgiving them for their trespassing, aren't you? And when you truly forgive yourself for your failings and shortcomings, are you not doing as the Bible suggests: loving your neighbour as *yourself*? Notice that this passage from the Bible hits upon both directions at the same time. It tells us to love others, but to love ourselves as well. It could also be translated into: blame not others as you would not blame yourself.

Every religion with which I am familiar makes a point of the human being's recognizing the fact that he is human, and that no amount of work or power can make him a god. In other words, all religions accept the fact that man is man, that he is weak, and that he will sin no matter how hard he tries not to sin. He may, of course, be able to reduce his objectionable behaviour considerably, but he will never stop it entirely. Man is not perfect, so he must act imperfectly. This means he will steal, cheat, hurt, be selfish, and so on. Only God is perfect, but he made us imperfectly. Therefore, he has the power of forgiveness regardless of what we have done. I know of no church that does not make total forgiveness by God one of its central beliefs.

The point I wish to make is that if God can forgive us our terrible behaviour shouldn't we be equally kind and generous with ourselves? Is it consistent with our religions to say, 'I know that God forgives me for my sins, but I can't'? This places our judgement above his. And this is the same point I have made from a psychological viewpoint. We need never blame ourselves for anything, because God made us imperfect. He knew he did it that way the moment he decided to do it, and he doesn't blame us for doing the stupid things that imperfect people are supposed to do.

If you follow these teachings from your religion or your Bible, I have no doubt you will seldom be depressed—at least not from self-blame. This is a perfect example where religion and psychology stand side by side and say almost the same thing. So don't feel guilty if you try to talk yourself out of feeling guilty the next time you misbehave. Remember, you are being unfaithful to your religion if you do feel guilt. It is hoped that you will admit *being* guilty as well as fight *feeling* guilty. You can do this without a sense of having betrayed your religious teachings. Even if your minister insists that you should feel worthless for an act you despise, tell him that he doesn't know his own teachings and hasn't the foggiest idea of what religion is supposed to be all about. The chances are that he gets depressed as often as you do because he thinks he is beyond redemption, and that he is totally unworthy because of some act for which he must hate himself for the rest of his life. When a minister gets emotionally upset, you can assume he hasn't followed his own religious teachings very well. Christianity and Judaism both have many wise statements, which, if interpreted correctly, can make one emotionally healthy for a lifetime. So, when a minister, or anyone else for that matter, is not emotionally stable he is not being true to his sacred teachings. I believe that all the essential points of a healthy psychology can be found in the Bible. The reason why so many people are disturbed, despite the fact that they are members of churches and have been all their lives, is that they read the messages incorrectly and therefore fail to lead truly exemplary lives.

My point is that you *are* likely to feel guilty if you do not suffer guilt over your misdeeds. You think that your religious teachings want you to suffer emotionally. You are wrong. Religion should not be a whip, it should be a blanket. If you get depressed, feel guilt, are overcome with fury, or are filled with fear, you are not being psychologically sound, but you are not being true to your faith either.

3

EMOTIONAL PROBLEMS

Assuming that you agree with me so far and would like to get rid of your burden of guilt, you will find that understanding much of what I've covered in Chapter 2 will give you some relief but not enough. To get over self-blame completely, you still need to know something about how all emotional disturbances are created and how each one of them can be eliminated.

Why You Really Get Upset

Most people think that we become disturbed in one of two ways. They believe that difficult circumstances or unhappy events make them disturbed. Or they think that someone who has something physically wrong with him cannot help being upset.

I personally think the major reason we get upset is that we talk ourselves into it! Our thoughts are the troublemakers, not our parents, husbands or wives, or bosses. It's not the puncture that gives you the fit of temper. It's the thoughts you have as you open the car door, put your foot out on the snow-covered road, and realize that you're going to have a rough time getting the tyre changed. It's the way we talk to ourselves that keeps us cool — or hot. This I call the ABC Theory of Emotions and goes like this: We can experience two kinds of pain. The first is a physical pain, and the other an emotional pain. If I throw a knife at your chest, and I call the knife A and the wound in your chest C, you will surely agree that A caused C, the knife caused the wound in the chest. Or if a car breaks your leg, the car is A and the broken leg C. The car broke your leg, or A caused C. This is always true of physical pain, even when you hurt yourself. Something has happened to your body which you can easily see and which comes usually from others. The skin is bruised, bones are broken, or blood is spilt.

Often we are in pain but cannot show any blood, broken bones, or bruised skin. Where does it come from? From B, the thoughts you have about A. It is your thinking that hurts you, not the things others have done or said to you. Suppose that someone calls you a foul name. The name-calling is A. You then tell yourself something like: 'Oh, isn't that dreadful, he doesn't like me. I can't stand it.' That is the sort of thing we all often do at B. The next thing we notice is a feeling of anger, or a headache, or a feeling of depression at C, in our bodies. We are inclined to think that the unpleasant words made us upset, when in fact it was our thinking about the words that hurt us. A does not cause us emotional pain, B does.

The thoughts that upset us at B are called irrational ideas. All of us have a number of irrational beliefs that cause us trouble, but we nevertheless believe in them very strongly. We have been so trained to think irrationally, stupidly, and nonsensically that it could come as a surprise, reading this book, to find out how much nonsense we hold sacred.

If you really want to stop being depressed, angry, or nervous, you will first have to see the sense of the idea that you always upset yourself. Then you will have to discover just what irrational ideas you are continually feeding yourself with. And finally you will have to come to understand that you have been taken in by stupid notions, and that you should replace this mental rubbish with more sensible ideas.

My point is that no one at any time, in any place can upset you in any way unless you allow it. Being imperfect, you naturally won't be able to fight your irrational tendencies all the time. But it's amazing how successful you can be if you know how you became upset and what you have to do to calm down. I've seen this work splendidly with scores of people who were disturbed most of their lives, but who then learned how to be largely undisturbed once they were shown how. But you must work very hard at changing your present thinking into sensible thinking. If you have happy thoughts, you will feel happy. If you have calm thoughts, you will feel unangry. And if you do not think fearful thoughts, nothing in the world is going to make you feel afraid.

In the past, we have always insisted that something or someone in our lives had to change if we were to become happier. This is wrong. Often those around us, or the situation in which we live, cannot or will not change. This need not condemn us to a life of misery. We can still manage successfully, even if the situation or the person in our life does not change. Thank God for small favours. Just imagine what living would be like if it weren't that way. It would mean that a woman with an alcoholic husband had no choice but to be depressed until he stopped drinking. And suppose he never stopped? She would have to be positively miserable all her life. That's nonsense. We *can* change for the better. All we need to do is change our thinking at B, and our feelings about A will change very dramatically at C.

The Irrational Ideas of the Self-blamer

Depression through self-blame is never caused because we have failed, because we have sinned, or because we accidentally hurt someone. Instead, self-blaming depression is caused at B because we believe that (1) we must be perfect or that (2) people are bad and should be severely blamed. These are two irrational ideas that always cause us to be depressed if we think of them and believe in them when we have done wrong.

I have explained in Chapter 2 why it is foolish to think that you have to be perfect and I have explained why you are never a bad person even though you have behaved badly. If you challenge these two ideas hard enough, you will find yourself level-headed and not at all depressed even when you're guilty of quite a number of misdeeds. But you must talk vigorously to yourself or it just won't work.

First, notice that you do indeed come up with these irrational beliefs just before you become depressed. If you don't notice it at first, slow down your thinking and try to catch yourself out. It may take some practice, but sooner or later you're almost certain to hear, loud and clear, some of the irrational things you have been saying at B for years.

A lady once came to me rather depressed after an argument with her husband. It seems that her husband would find a legitimate fault in her, she would argue in her defence but still wind up depressed. I suggested that she blamed herself over the real faults he pointed out because no one is any good unless they are faultless. At first she was not able to hear herself thinking these thoughts, but after several weeks she came to me saying: 'I'm beginning to see what you mean. All week I could suddenly hear myself saying the most awful things to myself. And they were all self-condemning things about myself. No wonder I get depressed.'

Don't be misled about these self-blaming thoughts. They always precede your feelings even if you can't recall a single thought you had before becoming depressed.

The fact that your mind may seem as though it's blank doesn't change anything. You *did* say something irrational to yourself if you now feel upset. Accept that on faith for the moment and then start practising listening to yourself *as* you get upset. Remember, your brain is never asleep even when you are. It is like the heart. It doesn't stop until you are dead.

Now, after you have convinced yourself that your moods come from your thinking, you must convince yourself next that that thinking really is wrong. To do this, you must do the same thing that you did when you got rid of your childhood superstitions. You once believed that black cats caused bad luck, that a broken mirror made your life miserable for seven years, and that dark rooms were dangerous because they were filled with ghosts. Do you believe in these superstitions today? I doubt it. Ask yourself the question, 'How did I rid myself of those beliefs even though most children believed the same nonsense?' You will discover that as you grew older you could think more clearly about ghosts and so on, and that you soon talked yourself out of those beliefs. Notice that you're not afraid of these things today because the ghosts have gone away or because you no longer break mirrors. And you still have cats crossing your path. In other words, A has not changed over the years. But C (your fears) has changed. Why? Obviously the only element that has changed is B − the way you think of A, that is, cats, mirrors, and ghosts. The moment you believed those beliefs were stupid beliefs, that was the moment you got rid of your fear. The change in attitude is the ingredient that brings this about.

How do we change our long-standing attitudes and beliefs? The same way that we changed our belief in Santa Claus. Only by thinking very carefully about

Santa Claus, by stopping to ask yourself how reasonable it is to think so-and-so. It was not simply a matter of your growing older that made you give up your belief in Santa Claus; it was your tendency to question as you grew older, along with the help of your friends who also questioned as they grew up. You must have asked yourself such questions as: 'How could Santa Claus get all the material he needed up there at the North Pole where there are no trees, no roads, no factories, and so on? How could he possibly make enough toys in one year to bring presents for all the children in the world? And if he is supposed to come down the chimney, what does he do if some are too small, or if a house doesn't have one at all? And wouldn't he be so filthy after a bit that the soot would choke him?' And so on and so on.

It is this kind of challenging and *nothing else* which changed your attitudes. Time has nothing directly to do with it, as you can clearly see if you go to the Caribbean islands where some people still stick pins into dolls to kill their enemies, and if you think how witchcraft is practised throughout the world. These people do not stop to analyse their beliefs, so they go on blindly believing in them.

It is through this same process that you have changed drastically some of the most forceful prejudices of childhood. Wasn't there a time when the thought of being naked before the opposite sex was shocking? Don't tell me that you don't undress before your spouse these days? Didn't you think that you wanted to be a cowboy or a fireman when you were a youngster but wouldn't think of it today? Haven't you changed your political views over the years? All these beliefs were held staunchly once upon a time but they changed over the years because you rethought them, analysed them, and seriously questioned them. *That* is what made them change. If you can rethink and question long-standing opinions, you can rethink and question the irrational teachings you were taught. All you have to do is think very thoroughly about the reasons you must be perfect, why everyone has to like you, or how can people really hurt you if they say unkind things to you. Think over those ideas and several others, throw them out or change them into sensible ideas, and you will rid yourself of more mental rubbish than you can believe.

How to Cope with Rejection

One of the reasons why people dread being rejected is their belief that the rejection means they're no good, that they wouldn't have been rejected if they'd been different, and that the rejection is proof of their worthlessness. According to this view, the person doing the rejecting is always right and superior, while the one rejected is always in the wrong and is somehow faulty.

But is this true? Why isn't there something wrong with the person who rejects me? Can't he be all screwed up and passing judgment on me based on his own weaknesses, jealousies, and prejudices? When you stop and realize that every single individual who ever lived and is living and will live is motivated by irrational feelings some of the time, how can you continue to think every judgement made by those irrational people out there must be accurate judgements? It seems to me this is the first lesson we must all make about the evaluations of others — others can be petty, prejudiced, mean, and envious. Their rejection of you tells you more about them than about yourself. For instance, if your friend goes to the greengrocer's and buys grapes, peaches, and bananas, but doesn't buy apples, what is he telling you about apples? That apples are bad? That no one else approves of apples? That apples should feel ashamed of themselves and break down and have a depression? Quite the contrary! Your friend's rejection of apples only tells us that *he* finds them distasteful and prefers other fruit. Other people will undoubtedly find these same apples quite satisfying. In short, you have learned a lot about your friend's *tastes* but nothing at all about apples.

And isn't it the same if your friend rejects you? He may not like your political views, but that hardly proves your views are wrong, does it? He may not like your looks any longer — perhaps your shoulder-length hair. Again, that says nothing about you, only about his prejudices. You might, of course, want to think over his views and decide whether he's right in his criticism and get your hair cut. But you could also decide he's wrong and let him go his way. Or if his friendship is very important to you, then cutting your hair to please him might be a sensible compromise with yourself, provided it wasn't that much of a sacrifice. In any event, his rejection of you might or might not be fair if you focus on the *thing* about you that he does not like. But it is never correct to conclude that his rejection of you is fair if he implies that you are a completely worthless human being. Even if everyone you know rejects you, that is still no proof of your lack of value as a human being. Thousands of people rejected Martin Luther King. Thousands rejected Jesus, for that matter. But this hardly means that these two men were bad or worthless.

Instead of being thrown off-balance by an occasional rejection, the wise person can try to win that approval back, or, if this seems pointless, he can accept the fact that he is only a human being who can never please everyone and set out to find people with whom he's compatible. This is particularly good advice where one's love life is concerned. I can't tell you how many people I have worked with who felt completely squashed just because someone they loved rejected them. Certainly, it's not nice to be disapproved of, but it's hardly life and death. In every case in which I've been successful in getting the rejected person to understand the reason for the rejection and asked him to improve that aspect of himself for which he was rejected (if it could be improved) and then urged him to find new people to relate to—in every case the rejection was soon forgotten or reduced in significance, or was used to good advantage, and other people were found with whom the individual got on quite well.

This is what I'm referring to when I say, 'Be kind to yourself.' Put yourself on a higher plane. Value yourself even if others don't, and you may be surprised how people will think more of you. Those people with a healthy sense of self-respect, who don't let an occasional rejection put them out, have fewer rejections to deal with than those who are always getting depressed because of a disapproval and who then try so hard to prevent the next rejection that they make too much effort to please others. They strain for approval and stand on their psychological heads to be loved. This will cool off more people than they ever suspect. People can sense when you are desperate for approval and it makes them uncomfortable. In addition, they wonder what's wrong with you that you have to try so hard to please them.

Expect Setbacks

As you come to understand what's depressing or disturbing you, there may be some improvement fairly quickly because you are trying hard, you are highly motivated, and you take up any advice that sounds as though it might help.

A second phase usually sets in at this point in which the old symptoms reappear and it seems as though no progress has been made. To understand these setbacks you must think of your behaviour as a complicated set of habits. You know how habits are. You don't need to think about them at all. You can drive your car through a town and have your thoughts on something else at the same time. Miles after leaving the town you wake up and wonder if you've come to that town yet. That is an example of how beautifully habits work for us.

Irrationally-motivated behaviour can be learned just as well, but the results of being controlled by irrational habits are much more unpleasant. Trying to change any habit usually requires great energy over a period of time and you must always expect failures. Making typing errors, smoking cigarettes, getting to bed late: these are all common habits and we all know how hard it can be to overcome them. Imagine how much more difficult it is to overcome a habit such as being afraid of people, remaining silent in a group, being lazy and skivving, running yourself down. Yes, these are habits too. And when you try to overcome them you can be sure you'll have plenty of lapses. That's to be expected. Habits can be overcome only through much work and after numerous failures. Remember the last part of that sentence. I once knew a man who misappropriated funds in the organization he worked for because he needed some ready cash and because it was a quick way to solve his problems. He also had a habit of lying his way out of a jam if he was questioned about his money-juggling. That was another bad habit. As such he should have expected that he would steal again and lie again even though he was seeking psychiatric help, and even though he had not done either of the above in months. Since it was a habit, there was every reason to believe that if he got into financial straits again, the habitual thing for him to do would be to embezzle money and wriggle and lie his way out of it.

This doesn't mean everyone has to repeat his symptoms after they are once under control. It only means that we get lazy about what we've learned and this permits the old habits to grow stronger over the days and weeks. And before we know it we have gone and done the wretched same thing again.

Be kind to yourself. Understand habits; their favourable and their unfavourable sides. And the next time you repeat some stupid action after you thought you'd got it taped, forgive yourself and realize how you were the victim of a habit. But then get going and fight the thing by thinking it out sensibly as you did before; the way that enabled you to gain the healthy control the first time.

It is also extremely important that people who are frustrated by the annoying behaviour of others understand all this. A husband who habitually comes home late for supper is certain to repeat this pattern even though after a quarrel he promises to improve, and yes, even though he has been doing better for a number of days. Habit is likely to have its way. If you kindly but firmly talk about the issue instead of fume over it, he can get quicker control over his habit the second time around; he won't be using his efforts to blame himself or you; and he can quietly analyse how the habit began to creep up on him again.

You Are Not Your Actions

One of the main reasons we have setbacks is that it is so easy for us to think of ourselves and our behaviour as being the same. Logical thinking practically seems to scream out that we must judge ourselves by our actions. It goes against everything that sounds reasonable not to value ourselves by our accomplishments, our financial successes, our conquests, and our popularity. So, when our behaviour is bad we are likely to feel the old irrational habit take hold and we have a setback.

Not valuing ourselves is such a difficult thing, however, that we should study the matter much more deeply so that we really understand the need to accept ourselves when we behave badly and talk ourselves out of the usual self-blame.

When you hate yourself because of some disagreeable act, you are actually making a number of rash statements. Suppose you say something offensive at a party and turn a few people against you. Among the thoughts you could and are likely to have are: 'Oh no! I spoke rudely to John.' (True.) 'I'm always saying stupid things just to get attention.' (False. No one always makes stupid or rude comments; only some of the time, and usually very infrequently at that.) 'I'll never learn to watch my tongue.' (False. How do you know what you will be doing in the future? What usually happens is that you believe you're the biggest fool in the place, and *then,* because you have convinced yourself of the hopelessness of it all, you fail to make the necessary effort to change, so you don't change. Then you pat yourself on the back for making so many correct predictions. You haven't predicted at all. You *forced* things to come out the way you convinced yourself they would come out.

So if you are not always being tactless, why should you hate yourself all the time? Before you made your rude remark, and after it too, you did a number of charitable things. You opened the car door for your wife. You helped your hostess with her chair at the dinner table. You drove the baby-sitter home that night. If bad actions make you bad, then shouldn't good actions make you good? If so, to find out if you are a decent human being or not, just keep a score each day and you will see that your kindnesses far outnumber your blunders.

At this point you're likely to protest that one can't exactly give oneself a medal just for opening a door for someone, or for taking home the baby-sitter. I disagree. Just stop and think for a moment what you'd think of your behaviour if you let the baby-sitter walk two miles home in the dark by herself. Wouldn't this be something you'd give yourself hell about? Then why not like yourself for doing a nice thing if you would definitely dislike yourself if you didn't do it?

The point I'm making is that most of the time you actually do behave decently, only you don't think about it. It is only when you behave less than perfectly that you take notice of your actions and get angry with yourself.

Perhaps another argument against judging yourself by your actions is the impossibility of describing you in your entirety as a person by a few unpleasant actions. If you are an alcoholic and cause trouble to others because of that, are we to believe that your alcoholic habit describes you completely? You are still supporting your family. You are honest in business. To say that all of you is worthless because part of you is deficient is like saying you should be shot if you have bad eyes, or stutter, or have a fear of lifts. Is a whole house worthless because the roof leaks? Is a new car ready for the scrap heap because it has a flat tyre?

No one in his right mind would hold such views. He would always separate the leak in the roof from the house as a whole. And he would immediately change the flat tyre rather than dump the car. In both instances the part would be separated from the whole and not used to describe the whole. It's the same with human beings. We all have faults and I refuse to believe I'm totally worthless just because parts of me are no good.

And lastly, even if you think your actions and you are the same, then why aren't the actions of children the same as the children? When a baby throws up on your lovely sofa you make one judgement about the vomiting and another judgement about the child (I hope). Don't tell me that you go around all day hating your children for the millions of irritating things they do. If you do, you are an ignorant and disturbed parent and are sure to raise problem children. But most of us have sense most of the time to separate the child from his behaviour and not judge him by his noise, disorder, mess, and fighting. We love him through the whole thing even though there is much at times we don't like about him.

If we think this is rational in the case of children, why should it be any different with adults? Because we, as adults, should know better? Of course not! That takes us back to the comments I have already made that we are not perfect because we are human and that we will all misbehave for reasons of stupidity, ignorance, or disturbance.

Learn How to Argue with Yourself

Some of my patients have been so brainwashed into believing their irrational beliefs that they find it terribly hard to talk and challenge themselves out of believing in all this nonsense. I've already explained to you the necessity of thinking about the reasonableness of your statements and shown you how you can change them if you analyse them carefully. Sometimes, however, more is needed. I can offer two other suggestions to help you change a sick attitude into a healthy one.

First, ask other people what they think about your beliefs. But make sure you put your questions mainly to those who are not bothered by the same kind of problems. If you ask a depressive how he deals with failure, you will only get back the same nonsense you've already been feeding to yourself, and that will tend to reinforce your irrational thinking, not weaken it. Instead, approach a few people who handle failure and depression better than you do and ask their thoughts on the matter. We are usually persuaded somewhat by the crowd, so use that power to help you over your problem. It's a strong weapon, because we are all influenced by group pressures to some degree. If most of your male friends are wearing flared trousers, you will almost certainly find yourself approving of them in time. The best example of group pressure I can think of, however, is this business of long hair. First the teenagers started it, then the younger adults picked it up, so did the entertainment people, and finally its influence was noticed even among M.P.s and in the business world.

So move in different circles, associate with those people who have the values which you want but which you haven't yet managed to adopt, and I assure you that some change in your thinking will probably follow.

The second important technique you can use to change your thinking, along with analysing your thinking, is to say the *rational* thought out loud (if you're alone), or think it to yourself if there are other people around. Even if you don't believe the thought, think it anyway. Before you can believe an idea it must at least be in your head. You must hear how it sounds to you.

Your irrational thought must be given some opposition even if it's half-hearted.

Haven't you ever tried on an article of clothing certain you wouldn't like it? No doubt you've done the same with food: you were sure you wouldn't like but you did once you tasted it a few times. And aren't there a number of people you learned to like, despite the fact you had an aversion toward them initially? You might have asked the Smiths over because the guests you really wanted were busy that weekend. And to your surprise you found some good qualities in the Smiths that you'd never have discovered had you not given them this half-hearted chance.

It's no different with our thoughts. If we try them on for size, we may be surprised how well they fit. So say sensible things to yourself when you're getting upset; even though you're not totally convinced by them. The next time you give yourself the works for making a mess of things fight those words with, 'No, I'm still acceptable to myself even if I wasn't perfect on the job.' You may then be inclined to say: 'Stop kidding yourself, you damn fool. You made a right royal mess and cost the company a packet. It would serve you right if you got the sack. Then whether you are able to believe yourself or not, say something like: 'I am not an idiot because I messed things up. Mistakes will happen and who knows, maybe I'll learn a lot from this mistake. Even if the company doesn't want me, *I* want me, I'm all I've got.' And so on. These sensible and charitable ideas may well begin to grow on you because you are *at least listening to them.* If you don't even give them that much of a chance, how ever do you expect to believe them at all?

The whole process will, or at least should, resemble an exciting debate. You take both sides. To begin with your irrational voice is louder and more convincing. At surface level, however, you are debating those long-held views in a less convincing voice. You must debate with yourself until the surface ideas grow in strength and replace the deeper ideas. When you utter an irrational belief, give it some opposition with a rational belief. Never let irrational beliefs go unchecked. Always give each of them an antagonist. Tit for tat. Spend as much time debating with yourself as you spend on blaming yourself and you'll be in clear water.

A further argument which you can always use to convince yourself that your irrational ideas deserve to be seriously debated is the fact that they are causing you trouble. Do you need more proof? If your ideas and beliefs were so sound, why would you be reading this book? If you are such a wonderful example of Mr or Mrs Average-Normal, then how is it you get so depressed, or worried, or hostile at times? Like it or not, your present methods just aren't working or you would be feeling splendid most of the time. If you are in some kind of emotional turmoil most of the time, then don't tell *me* how right and proper your attitudes and philosophies are. If they don't work for you, why should they work for me?

To sum up, I urge you to say the proper thoughts to yourself even if you do not believe them. That shows you to be reasonably receptive to new possibilities, and from there who knows how far you can go? Only by following this advice will you ever be able to accept such revolutionary ideas as: there are no bad people in the world, only bad deeds; no one can upset us emotionally, only physically; everyone has the right to be wrong and should not be condemned for his wrongdoing; and so on. Work at it and make it work!

4
SELF-PITY

If you have ever felt sorry for yourself, you are already familiar with the second major cause of depression: self-pity. Strange as it may seem, this can crush you every bit as badly as guilt can. You can't tell by looking at a depressed person in which way he is depressing himself. The reasons for feeling wretchedly miserable can be as different as night from day, but the end result is practically the same. Only in its extreme form does depression from guilt really take on a different character from depression by other means. For example, extreme guilt reactions sometimes cause people to punish themselves with knives, razor blades, cigarettes, etc., something not usually seen in the other forms of depression.

If you suspect you might be a self-pitier, face it. Too many people feel so guilty about being self-pitiers they never get an insight into their own motives and the forces which act on them. I suppose the reason is that self-pity is associated with immaturity, the childish manipulation of others, and takes on the characteristics of the hysterical woman.

Be that as it may, it's still in your best interests to consider the possibility that you mope around all the time because you feel sorry for yourself. If you can't persuade yourself you are blaming yourself for something or that you are breaking your heart over someone else's troubles, then you can be reasonably sure that you're pitying yourself. Hard medicine to swallow perhaps! If you fight this insight, you will simply get nowhere. You will waste your time or the time of whoever is trying to help you much as one of my patients once did because she simply could never face the fact that she was a first-class self-pitier. I constantly agreed with her that she had suffered a most unfortunate setback to her family life and I agreed there was no rational reason why in heaven's name it should have happened to someone like her. She had always lived a life above suspicion, been charitable to all, harmed no one, and then her fiancé and favourite sister died within six months of each other.

There was no reason why she should have felt guilty over these events, and although she was partly depressed over feeling sorry for the deceased, she could easily see that they were beyond suffering and safely in heaven. So that could not have been the major reason for her lengthy and deep feelings of despair. When I suggested that she felt sorry for herself because this stinking world had treated her so unfairly, she protested so vigorously I was actually taken aback. I had never seen such unwillingness to consider oneself a self-pitier. This observation, and many more of a similar nature, has led me to conclude that if you are not sure how you are depressing yourself, take a guess and look at self-pity very closely.

Two Thoughts Which Bring On Self-pity

Whenever you attempt to understand your self-pitying moods always ask yourself what you were thinking of immediately before you became upset. Then, of all the thoughts you can recollect, analyse and sort out those which make sense and those which do not. If you do this properly, you will practically always come to the point where you have made the following two statements over some issue or event in your life: (a) I want my way in this matter and (b) it's awful if I don't get my way.

The first thought is a reasonable one and can never cause you any serious harm. As long as you want, desire, prefer, or wish for anything, you will never be upset if you don't get what you desire. All of us have already wished for a million things we haven't received and it hasn't hurt one bit even though it may have left a rather saddened feeling. Haven't you ever wanted to be a film star, to be rich, to be famous, to write *the* great book, or to be the world's champion belly dancer? And hasn't this been a pleasant daydream even though it never seems to come true? As long as you take these wishes with a pinch of salt you won't get depressed if they don't materialize. It's only when you think that you *must* be right, when you believe it's the *end of the world* not to have your dream yacht on the Mediterranean, that you begin to be upset.

Understand this thoroughly: you do not *need* a great deal in this life, and in fact you do not even *need* to live. Let's look at that first thought. All you need for life is food, shelter, and clothing. More than this makes living very nice but is hardly essential. It's wonderful to have friends, but you will not die if you do not have them. You could always become a hermit. However, it is unlikely you'll ever have to go that far because there will always be someone around who'll sell you some bread and rent you a room. You could die without the bread or the room, but you certainly are not going to die if you break up with one or more of your close friends. What you do have to be careful of is that people don't *hate* you so very much that they are likely to shoot you in the street or not sell you food, etc. It's people's hatred, not their love, you should be *very* much concerned with.

The second thought, that you do not need to live, is easily proved when you stop to think of the numerous instances when you would voluntarily sacrifice your life for someone you loved or didn't even know. You would risk your life for your family, for your country, for someone who seemed to be drowning, or for someone in a burning building calling for help. Countless heroic acts have been performed by people who obviously believed that they didn't consider life all that essential or they would never have risked it. Yet these same people might have been depressed the previous day because they thought it was the end of the world when their jobs folded or when they were told they had cancer.

Distinguishing Between Sadness and Tragedy

Another way of looking at these ideas is to see them as a confusion between what you think of as being sad and what you think of as being tragic. There are a great many events in your life that are sad, but only a few of them are tragic (even here, many tragedies would not hit you so hard if you viewed them differently).

Sad things give us feelings of regret and disappointment. These are not devastating emotions. We experience them often, with no ill effects, and they often don't last very long. But tragedies are a different matter. When we believe we've been stricken with a catastrophe we usually can't respond calmly to it.

Most of our self-pitying depression comes because we confuse sad things with catastrophic or tragic events. That is, we honestly believe that what we're experiencing is *awful*, the *end of the world*, and simply *unbearable*. But is it? Where's the proof that something is awful? Who says it is? If you didn't listen to the sympathetic commiseration of your well-meaning friends, or to your own declarations of disaster, do you suppose for a minute you'd be so upset? Not in a thousand years. You have to *talk* yourself into thinking that an event is unbearable, and most of the time (about ninety-nine percent) you're quite wrong. The great majority of events in our lives are regrettable, not terrible; are disappointing, not catastrophic; are sad, not tragic. If we unthinkingly talk or think ourselves into believing that something is terrible, catastrophic, or tragic, we will, in the immediate moments following this kind of thinking, become low-spirited. But if we see clearly that so many things which happen to us are only regrettable, disappointing, and sad, we will simply be mildly unhappy for a short time and then come back to a normal and optimistic mood.

Jim returned from the college dance with his steady girl friend only to be told by her that she wanted to break up. He immediately went downhill and called in to see me the next day, very depressed. After hearing the facts, I could easily determine that something *sad* had happened to the young man (his girl friend was rejecting him) and that he had reacted to this surprising news by making a tragedy out of it (I'll die if I can't have her love).

I managed to show Jim very quickly how he was pitying himself and what he would have to do to stop this depression.

'It isn't because your girl friend is rejecting you that you're so down-hearted, Jim,' I protested. 'It's because you think it's awful to be rejected.'

'But it is. I didn't sleep all night wondering what I had done to make her turn against me and wondering what I would do from now on.'

'No, Jim, that's not why you're upset. The way you explained your relationship with your girl friend made good sense. You can't get depressed by trying to learn from your mistakes. Self-pity only comes when you think you *must* have something and that it's terrible and unbearable if you don't get it. In this case you were telling yourself that you still wanted to be close to the girl, and had you stopped there, you would have felt just sad and nothing more. But you went further and convinced yourself that being rejected was unfair, that it was a terrible thing to do after all you had done for her, and that why did this lousy business have to happen to you anyway. When you believed these last ideas you wound up by eating your heart out and silently saying "Poor me".'

'But I knocked myself out for her, and now to be treated this way is very unfair.'

'Yes it's unfair, but why shouldn't it be? Just because you don't want unfair things to happen to you does that mean they can't? Is it the end of the world just because you didn't get your way? Why couldn't you learn from this experience, consider it a pleasant memory, and go forth and woo a dozen new girl friends? You could do that fairly easily if you'd stop pitying yourself because she dumped you.'

And so it went on for sometime until he could see how he'd made a mountain out of a molehill. The next time I saw him a week later he was completely over the bad patch and taking another girl out! I attributed his change to the fact that he easily saw how he had convinced himself that a sad event is no different from a tragic event. It is a lesson every self-pitier must learn if he cares about his mental health.

Disturbances Are Worse than Frustrations

Life is an endless series of frustrations. No one can go through even so much as one day without being somewhat frustrated (not having everything his own way). The only people who do not experience frustrations are up in heaven or in the grave. The rest of us in the land of the living cannot escape frustrations any more than we can escape illness, taxes, or death. To be alive means to be frustrated. Therefore, to seek a life without frustration is like asking to die. So let's be satisfied to have these constant pains in the neck but learn at last how to swim with the tides.

If you don't distinguish between frustrations and disturbances, you will do two things that can harm you badly. On the one hand, you will be making matters infinitely worse by adding the pain of the disturbance to the pain of the frustration, and on the other hand, you will be so mixed up from the disturbance you won't be able to work out a way to remove the frustration.

Take the case of Fred, a once-popular boy until he went off to university. His acquaintances there didn't know he was such a whizzkid, so they treated him like the rank and file instead of as a leader. This undermined his confidence badly, and Fred soon felt so sorry for himself that he became depressed. He began to doubt his own worth and was soon keeping to himself. The lack of recognition naturally continued until Fred took an overdose of drugs and nearly died. This brought him into the limelight immediately and for a while he was the talk of the faculty. But even this petered out in a matter of days and left Fred unrecognized once more. Again he turned this into a catastrophe and thought he had to do something desperate to catch the attention of the place. So Fred deliberately got drunk and had an accident. His name was read out on the TV news, and his arrest was the talk of the university for a while. When the dust settled and Fred was back at lectures he found things worse than ever. By now his associates had sized him up as a freak and had even less to do with him than before. After a couple of other attention-getting accidents, Fred decided he had had it and thought it was time to get some help. Not only was he still lonely and depressed but he had lost time and missed valuable lectures, had injured himself several times, and had collected a police record to boot.

This is what I mean by a disturbance being worse than a frustration. Had Fred not made so much of being an unknown student and had he allowed his normal talents to thrust him forward into the notice of other students, he could eventually have regained a position of prestige and leadership. Instead, Fred believed that to be unknown was a fate worse than death, that he simply could not stand being unpopular, and that any course of action was justified to correct this frustration. So he proceeded to hurt himself infinitely more than his unpopularity was hurting him. In addition, while he was in the grips of this irrational belief, he was actually unable to see how he was making matters worse and how, by changing just a few moves in his strategy, he could get practically all he wanted. However, a disturbed mind does not think in clear terms, so Fred went from bad to worse until he sought help and found out how he was incorrectly believing that not being a leader at university was terrible, that he ought to feel sorry for himself and get everyone else to feel the same way, and that being frustrated was the worst of all fates, even worse than being upset.

Self-pity from False Accusations

Most people take criticism very badly. They feel so hurt and lose so much sleep over the unkind remarks and insults of others that a thorough knowledge of how to handle this situation is needed if they are going to keep their wits about them and avoid another occasion for being wretched.

The next time you're accused of anything, you can avoid being disturbed over it if you will ask yourself two questions: 'Is it true?' or, 'Is it false?' If you decide that it's true, don't blame yourself for being found guilty, since as a human being you have the right to be at fault. Suppose your husband calls you a tart because you enjoy dancing with other men at parties. You mingle freely among the guests but he insists you are flirting, and he insists you stop. Instead of pitying yourself for being so misunderstood, simply examine his statement carefully and decide whether he is right or wrong.

Suppose you decide he's right. Well and good. You have been a flirt. You have enjoyed leading the men on and you honestly have to agree that you would be very upset indeed if your husband behaved as you do at parties. Now you have to convince yourself that you are not an evil person merely because you were thoughtless. You have a right to be wrong, and in fact you are grateful for your husband's telling you that your behaviour looks over-free, because you can then change it. Since you don't want to make such an unflattering impression at parties, you will try very hard to avoid this pattern in the future.

Notice how you've profited from being called a tart instead of allowing yourself to become depressed? Quite an improvement, wouldn't you say?

Now suppose that after thinking over his accusation carefully you decide he's totally wrong. Why should you be disturbed over this? It's really only a matter of his opinion against yours. You surely don't become disturbed over every difference of opinion that you two have, so why should you make this an exception merely because you are now disagreeing about you? You need only tell yourself: 'There he goes again, the poor dear. Every time I dance with another man he makes himself insensibly angry because he thinks I'm going to have an affair with every man I touch. I wonder what *his* problem is? Maybe he has too little confidence in his ability to keep me and that's why he gets so worried when I'm not there beside him at all times. Well, that's his problem. He can't help it, and I certainly didn't create it for him, so why should I get all hot and bothered because he thinks I'm a tart? I'm not one and if he thinks I am, he'll just have to decide what he wants to do about it.'

It makes no difference what the accusation is. It can always be handled in a kindly and charitable way towards the person making the unkind remark if you always keep the above facts in mind. This also means that no one can insult you. No matter what they say about you, all you have to do to take the sting out of the remark is ask yourself whether the remark is true or false. An insult is something we do to ourselves. It is not something done to us by others. What they do is give us their opinions; what we do is make something personal out of it and get all insulted that others should have ideas in their heads that we disapprove of.

Recently a patient of mine said she had been highly insulted the previous night because a man propositioned her rather brazenly in the presence of her husband. Needless to say, the husband was incensed and ready for a fight. But I insisted they had insulted themselves and that they needn't have taken the man's remarks so personally. For one thing, she was probably not the only woman he ever thought of propositioning, so why should she think it was only she that he was singling out? Secondly, he was really being flattering to make such a suggestion, since there are probably many women he would never think of asking for such favours. Thirdly, was he actually hurting anyone with his crude ways? The poor fool must have been terribly insensitive to make such a faux pas in the first place, or he must have been terribly lonely and desperate to come on like a bull in a china shop. One should have sympathy and compassion for anyone who is that miserable inside. And instead of taking a swing at the bloke or feeling insulted, how much more sensible it would have been for my patient to say, 'No thanks,' to the man, that she appreciated his kind thought and that her husband must surely be flattered by it as well. She could have ended by wishing him good hunting! Wouldn't that have been an achievement?

Avoiding Depression Over an Unfaithful Spouse

There are generally two typical reactions to the discovery that your spouse has committed adultery. The first is that you have let your partner down and you feel terribly guilty about it. The second is self-pity because you don't know how you could be treated so shabbily after all the sacrifices you made for your beloved. Of course, after either of these initial reactions subsides, there is an upsurge of resentment and bitterness that can get amazingly furious.

I suggest that if you behave in either of these ways you are being just plain silly and should seriously consider facing such an event in something like the following manner.

Be grateful that it was not you who had to resort to an affair. You at least had the willpower and fortitude to resist a flirtation, while your impulsive and dependent spouse could not do so. Aren't you proud of yourself for this accomplishment? And don't you have compassion for your lover because he or she could not resist temptation? Yes, take pride in your superior control. Remaining loyal isn't the easiest thing in the world to do by any means, especially these days. To keep your wedding vows takes a fortitude not many people have.

What you have to see is that both of you had thought of having affairs many, many times, and both of you had many opportunities to do so, but you were mature enough to stick by your promises. You showed your capacity for dependability and trust while your spouse failed in both of these vital areas of married life.

And if your spouse comes back at you with: 'But I wouldn't have looked for an affair if you had only done this or that for me. It's your fault I was driven into someone else's arms.' Don't swallow that stuff. Any day of the week you could pull out a list of complaints against your mate that can match his list against you. Still you did not let these grievances throw *you* off the path. You took him with all the faults and worked around them. You didn't use them as excuses for holding hands with someone in the back row of the cinema.

When you look at infidelity this way you will feel pride in yourself and compassion for your mate. You certainly can't feel depressed (*a*) if you aren't blaming yourself for not being the perfect mate and (*b*) if you aren't convincing yourself the sky has fallen in. An affair is usually nothing more than a serious message that something is wrong in the marriage. That something need not always be you. It could just as well be the partner.

One patient of mine I shall never forget had affairs for years and his wife knew it. She cursed herself that he always had to run around with other women, thinking he was doing this because she was seriously lacking in something as a woman. When she came to me she was quite depressed and had as low an opinion of herself as one can have. But all this changed when I convinced her that her husband ran around because he was a human alley cat and no matter what kind of wife she was it would never keep him at home for long. I told him this one day when both of them came to see me together and after a moment's thought he had to admit that it was absolutely true because he really could not find serious fault with his wife. In fact, the idea struck him as rather startling, so he eventually decided to divorce his wife and be honest with her for the first time in years. He simply liked alley catting around and had no intention of stopping. What he wanted from marriage was a maid, a cook, and a laundress. He decided that this was unfair to his wife, so he let her go to find another man who would love her only.

Neurotics Often Slip

To spare you a lot of depression if you have a habit of pitying yourself, remember always that the behaviour of others changes in a very uneven way. One day a person behaves admirably and maturely and then the next day is right back to the same old tricks. This can be exasperating after you have not seen the annoying behaviour for quite a while and you think that at last the person has conquered it.

If you are finally at peace with yourself because your child has stopped stealing, brace yourself. If the right pressures come together, he can begin stealing again as though he had never had any help and as though you had never made any dent in his pattern. If you are not careful at such moments, you are likely to throw up your hands in desperation and make a catastrophe out of how futile all your efforts have been and how you might just as well throw in the sponge.

This would be a serious mistake. This is not the time to get depressed. Remember that anything we learn tends to be forgotten with time. This applies to our behaviour just as well as it does to the multiplication table. People get sloppy in their thinking if they aren't practising rational thoughts. That's why an ex-alcoholic can start drinking all over again. That's why a child who hasn't stolen anything for six months can suddenly start again. And that's why you too can get depressed again even though you thought you understood how you get that way and haven't been really low-spirited for a year. When we drop our guard we ask for trouble.

It is no different from dieting. Suppose that you came to me to lose weight and you learned to discipline yourself so well that you took off all the weight you wanted. Would that be the end of the story? Would that mean you didn't have to diet and fight temptation constantly from then on? Of course it wouldn't. To keep the weight off, you would have to diet practically every day for the rest of your life. To remain undisturbed you must watch yourself or you will find yourself being angry, down-hearted, or fearful. And to get out of that mood you would have to do the same things you did to gain calmness before.

A slip is hardly an awful thing and surely doesn't mean that no gains have been made at all. Gains are measured in three ways: frequency, duration, and severity.

Frequency: if your husband is now quarrelling with you only once a week whereas before he was doing so every day, he has made a significant gain. Be happy!

Duration: if his arguments last only an hour instead of all night, he has made a gain. Be happy!

Severity: if he only throws cups and saucers instead of putting his fist through the wall, he has made a gain. Be happy!

The idea that our cranky behaviour will automatically stop when we've uncovered a long-forgotten memory which has supposedly been eating at our unconscious ever since childhood is Freudian mythology. Sometimes behaviour does stop wonderfully abruptly, but in the majority of cases it diminishes slowly, fading out gradually. Woe to the person who expects a flash of insight to make one's spouse or child wake up a new person. That individual is doomed to depression.

Self-pity Can Be a Powerful Weapon

Because practically everyone believes that he can be made upset by others or that he can upset others, it has occurred to millions of people to use this observation in controlling people. One of the best ways to control others is through guilt. If you show your friend how hurt you are because of something she said, you are hoping she will feel bad about her remark and never treat you like that again. One sure way to convince her that she is really mean for what she did is to make a long face, cry a bit, and hope your self-pity crushes her. In all likelihood you will achieve your aim beautifully, since your friend will certainly blame herself for making you so miserable.

This is a favourite technique of control used by possessive mothers to keep their children from growing up. 'Come home by eleven, Jenny,' the mother says to her adult daughter. 'You know how worried I get when you're not in. I can't sleep a wink while you're out.'

Mamma wants Jenny to see her pain. That is what will bring Jenny home. If Jenny had any sense, she would say to her mother: 'I hope you won't worry about me, Mother. But if you insist on making yourself all nervous and depressed over my not being in early, then I suppose you'll just have to worry. You're the one who is upsetting you, not me. If that problem bothers you a great deal, I hope you'll do something about it.'

I know a great many readers will protest that this is unkind treatment of the mother, totally devoid of respect for her tender concern. On the contrary. For Jenny to do otherwise is tantamount to making a worrier and a depressive out of her mother. The more the girl accepts the responsibility for the mother's disturbance, the more the mother will tend to use her grief and anguish to get her way. How kind is that?

One of the most powerful ways in which self-pity is used is as a suicidal threat. When your boyfriend says to you, 'Sally, marry me or I'll kill myself,' he is feeling so sorry for himself that he hopes you'll take pity on him and agree to the marriage. The sorrier he feels, the better a chance he usually has for getting his way with those people who have a soft spot in their hearts for martyrs. The dangerous part of this practice is the fact that responding to this pity encourages it all the more. This could lead to further suicidal threats and perhaps eventually to a successful suicide!

No one knows just how many drug users and alcoholics get started on their habits out of a feeling of self-pity, but I would guess that the percentage is staggering and is much more than most authorities appreciate. I can speak more knowledgeably about alcoholics than addicts and in that area I am sure a great deal of drunkenness is for nothing else than to make someone feel guilty or sorry.

Just listen to a crowd of men at a bar now and then: you'll hear all the self-pitying nonsense you can possibly stomach. A man may get drunk because the little woman was irritable or because she paid more attention to the dog than to him. Whatever the reason, it's fair to state that drinkers are not only a sorrowful lot, but usually feel sorry for themselves as well.

I don't wish to demean or be harsh on alcoholics, but

I think the truth hurts less than ignorance. So let me say this: alcoholics and heavy drinkers are very often insecure individuals who cry in their beer because they don't get their way. Ever noticed a child when he doesn't get what he wants? He often makes a play of being so upset one would think the world was coming to an end. To see what he goes through, you'd think going to bed early was going to kill him. All the tears and screaming is self-pity, pure and simple, and it has one purpose: to work on *your* sense of pity for him so that you'll give in.

What is involved in this situation is not only self-pity but other-pity as well. I shall be dealing with that in more detail in the next chapter, but for the present it is important to realize what power you give to others by giving into their self-pity techniques. I can think of a score of patients who have never grown up because they were such successful sympathy seekers. Why learn to accept things philosophically when all it takes to get your way is to appear crushed, scream your head off, show people what anguish you're in, and then keep this up until they say they're sorry?

I was reminded again recently just how deliberate all these self-pitying hysterics can really be. One young man rang me up and talked for half an hour. He was as cool and collected as you please, made sense, and for all the world seemed to be on top of things. A couple of hours later his father rang from the local psychiatric ward to tell me that the young man was lying profusely and that I hadn't the foggiest notion of what was really happening to his son. It seems that only minutes after the son rang me, he had had a wild scene at home during which he behaved so oddly and so tempestously it was thought advisable to take him to hospital. Before agreeing to enter, however, he wanted to ring me up for advice.

Again I was talking to the calmest, most contained, and sensible person I had talked to all day.

What was happening, of course, was the calculated use by the boy of throwing an emotional fit merely to get sympathy and to force his parents to be so worried that they would be too scared to do anything drastic. Little did they realize how they were being sucked into his little game which in this instance backfired a little bit.

Protecting Yourself from Becoming a Doormat

One of the unhealthiest consequences of pitying your-sels is that you will allow people to use you, manipulate you, and take advantage of you. Countless millions of children and adults go through their lives licking their wounds, suffering in silence, crying in privacy, and feeling that they have no right to stand up for themselves.

The self-pitier goes along thinking he has no rights, believing that a confrontation with his spouse is worse than having high blood pressure or migraine headaches, and feeling for some mysterious reason that he must always be wrong whenever someone challenges his think-ing. Underlying this sad state of affairs is a fear of think-well of oneself, a fear of being selfish and self-centered. And there is some truth to this. But one must under-stand what is meant by selfishness. I regard some selfish-ness as perfectly sane and healthy. I don't like the use of the word 'selfish,' because it suggests wanting one's own way exclusively. That's an immature way to live and hardly worth recommending. But if we change the word and call it 'enlightened self-interest,' then we come closer to what all healthy people possess.

Look around you now and then and notice how the strong people in your life, in politics, where you work, all have a high degree of self-interest. They do not mind in the least standing up for their rights, arguing at some length if necessary, and breaking up relationships if that is what is called for. They don't let themselves be pushed around, because they don't feel sorry for themselves when injured. Instead, they feel indignant and immediately become assertive because *fair* is *fair*. This is the key to overcoming your tendency toward becoming a doormat. When you really feel you have been fair in your dealings, don't give very much more or you will find yourself feeling abused and unappreciated. Some people just aren't going to play fair, because they honestly don't see what you are so unhappy about. You must tell them or write it out for them, or perhaps even show in your actions that you've had enough. Unless you do this, you will pity yourself, get depressed, and make your friend or spouse feel guilty or angry. You could, of course, continue your self-pity and carry it to extremes to get your way, but just think what it would cost you to win this way. Generally what happens when your self-pity doesn't work is that you finally have a confrontation, and for a time there is a change. As the days go by, however, there's a gradual re-establishment of the old pattern where you do all the dishes, spend evenings at home alone while he is out with the boys, and so on.

To avoid this trap, remember that *no one steps on you without your allowing it.* You actually co-operate in a person's controlling you. The fact that you often complain and cause minor changes to be made does not change the fact that eventually things fall into their old pattern because you allow them to.

This happens because (*a*) you think too little of yourself, (*b*) you will do too much to preserve a relationship, since you think you will never get another one, or (*c*) both. Then the only thing you have left is the strangely dissatisfying feeling that no one understands you, that you will just have to suffer through life while others get their way, and that maybe somewhere in heaven they have a very special place for martyrs.

Enough of this! The time has come for you to let those around you know once and for all that you have had enough of their pushing you around and unless they give up at once they will no longer get your co-operation, and if need be, the relationship will dissolve. It might amaze you how quickly most people will start giving in when they see that you really won't be bamboozled any longer.

I shall never forget the case of the mouse that roared. Ruth was a sheepish and bedraggled young divorcée. Her three children were her total responsibility and she was trying to do a proper job of bringing them up, but she lived near her mother and sister. A boyfriend or two also entered the picture from time to time. Between these people and Ruth there was usually the most lop-sided relationship I had ever seen. Ruth simply couldn't say, 'No'. Or rather, she *wouldn't* say, 'No'. Whatever her mother or sister asked of her she did. It mattered not that Ruth had work planned, or that she was tired running her own household, or that she needed help from others. All they had to do was suggest a favour and Ruth felt obliged to jump to it and help out.

She kept her resentment to herself all through these episodes and wouldn't do anything to let the others know how fed up she was. Naturally, in time she became quite depressed. When I saw her she looked like gloom itself. So I immediately tried to show her that being bossed by everyone was something she allowed because she was afraid of being rejected and afraid of hurting their feelings. I explained how rejection itself did not hurt people unless they made a big thing of it, and hurting other people's feelings was impossible unless *they* allowed themselves to be hurt. I suggested that, instead of feeling sorry for herself because others could not see their unfairness, Ruth start by being fair to herself first and to let the dust settle as it may. If her sister or her mother disowned her for her independence, she would at least get them off her back, a not inconsequential relief. In all likelihood, however, I suspected that the more respect Ruth showed herself, the more respect she would gain from others.

The very next week she came to me to report she had turned down her sister's telephone request to baby-sit. It was difficult for her to do and she was quite nervous as she stood up for herself for the first time in years, but she stuck to her guns and politely hung up the phone. For the next few hours she was jittery and unsure of herself, but she also had a new sense of strength. Whatever the new feeling was that was coming over her it was delicious, and on hearing her describe it, I knew she was experiencing the lifting of her depression.

Armed with this experience she next faced her mother, and the same emotional reactions followed. From her mother she transferred this technique to the butcher. Not getting a good cut of meat one day, she took it back and insisted on another cut worth the money she had spent on it. And so it went on. The mouse in her had died and so had the depression. Ruth was never the same after that. In addition to this new-found self-respect, she saw a marked change in the degree of respect she now received from other people. They no longer automatically told her what she should do, they asked most politely. And if Ruth was able to do the favour, she did so gladly. If not, she refused and that was that. The smile on her face, the lilt in her step, and the lively look on her face clearly indicated that the doormat was talking back.

If you are a doormat or a mouse, then think over very carefully why you can't stand rejection, and think over very carefully whether your standing up for yourself causes people their disturbances. Unless you see these two pieces of nonsense for what they are, you will never break free and be yourself. The result will be abuse, contempt, and domination by others, and depression for yourself.

When to Give In

Since self-pity is often a matter of giving in too constantly to others, the question naturally arises, 'When should I give in and when should I stand my ground?'

The answer is fairly simple. Give in on issues that matter very little to you. Stand your ground on issues that matter a great deal. Sometimes you may be able to live with a compromise and sometimes you may not be able to do so. Follow your feelings in this respect.

The only weakness in this advice is in the difficulty most people have of deciding what is really important. I suppose the best way to gauge this is to ask yourself whether you can live with the frustration gracefully or whether you will find yourself becoming more and more bitter about giving in until you finally have to explode.

Martha hated to make an issue with her husband about his being so slow when she waited to pick him up after work. He often let her wait far beyond any reasonable time she thought he would really need. But because she didn't want to rock the boat she didn't say anything or make a big scene. So she tolerated her husband's thoughtlessness for months, all the while getting more and more peeved, until one day she tore such a strip off the poor man he was absolutely speechless. She felt so bad about this loss of control that she apologized the next day and went right back to waiting for him while he loitered and she sat. No longer did she feel she had a right to make an issue out of it, because after all, what is so awful about having to wait thirty to sixty minutes for your husband if it keeps peace in the family and keeps the marriage together?

Martha would have been so much more sensible to recognize her true feelings: she detested waiting and felt that her husband had no reason whatever for fiddling around in the shop while she was sitting out in the hot sun or the freezing winter. The number of depressions she could have spared herself are countless. All she had to do was realize she was irritated by this unthinking behaviour and even though she could ignore it for a while she was sure to say something about it in the long run. And that was the key to her making up her mind. If she thought she could not keep her mouth shut indefinitely about his behaviour, then the sooner she spoke up about it the better. At least that way he would know immediately where he stood; she would feel better immediately because she had got her grievance off her chest; and lastly, because the complaint was registered early enough it would never become a vicious attack.

Martha could have had one more set-to with her husband, warned him that she would drive off if he were not out in the car after five minutes past closing time, and then do precisely that. In no more than one or two instances would he have clearly seen how important this issue was to his wife and he probably would have jumped to it. It is what we do about what we say we will do that counts, not what we say we will do. Or, to be trite, actions speak louder than words, and no more is this true than in this sort of situation.

Let us review this matter once more. Waiting for a late husband may not be a big thing with you, but it was for Martha. Therefore, it was her obligation to herself, and to her husband, to do something about it. She, furthermore, knew it was more than merely a passing annoyance by the fact that she could not overlook it. If she could not overlook it, she should then deal with it, and the sooner the better. For her, waiting in the car was, therefore, not something she should have given in to. She might not have minded it if her husband had walked out on her; in that case she could have accepted his running around philosophically. Another woman might not have accepted that with tranquility. So be it! To each his own. Only be true to yourself and recognize what you will tolerate and what you won't. Then either ignore it for good or do something about it the very next time it comes up.

Is Violence Ever Justified?

You may now be wondering if physical blows are included in my belief that one has a right to stand up for oneself. Damned right! But only in self-defense. Hitting people (children excluded) should be limited only to those rare occasions where one might be harmed. I see no other reason for harming adults, and I also cannot see any good coming out of a beating under any other circumstances.

There is an even better reason for not resorting to violence. To avoid being manipulated, you need only refuse to co-operate with the person trying to control you. You do not have to sneak up on him and pound him over the head with a rolling pin while he sleeps. That kind of behaviour can get you a life sentence at the most, and an excellent enemy at the very least. You are also likely to get a pounding yourself one day if you use that solution.

A better method to avoid being controlled is to refuse to co-operate with your controller. For instance, the wife of a jealous husband can allow herself to be dictated to and remain home to avoid an argument because Roger thinks she is going to hold hands with every third man she meets. If she does this, she will stop enjoying herself by not getting out of the house. Then she will feel sorry for herself, and presto, she is depressed.

Or, she can tell him sweetly that she is going to bingo with a few of the girls. And if Roger starts shoving her around, she should fight back. He started using violence, so she has a right to fight back. However, if she weighs only 9½ stone and he weighs 13 stone and is also a karate black, belt champion, she would be a fool to defend herself that way. But she could call the police later, or she could divorce him unless he saw her right to be free and go out when she wanted. Having some time to herself and going where she wants is a right she has as an adult. If she gives in on this issue, she will make a dictator out of her husband. So she might just as well let him know in no uncertain terms what aggression is going to accomplish for the male chauvinist pig!

It may seem to some of you readers that I am taking a rather hard stand. Such is not the case. I'm only suggesting that people who are controlled by others usually get their fill of it sooner or later, and if they act sooner, they spare themselves a lot of grief. I have known any number of women who for years excused their cowardice with all sorts of rationalizations: 'I'd get hurt'. 'The children need a father.' 'How could I manage alone?' But when the day comes on which she cannot take his bullying any longer, all those excuses go out of the window, and suddenly our sweet, cowardly, and scared rabbit of a wife finds the strength to face Mr Bully. The sad thing about her action is the fact that it came so late. Some women don't get up enough gumption until they've suffered abuse from their children, employers, or husbands for twenty years. They don't realize that they have a breaking point, that that point will be reached some day, so why not do something about it early and avoid years of suffering?

Only Lions Love Martyrs

One of the last things I want to say about self-pity is that it often backfires and turns people *against* you whom you so desperately want to be *for* you. The truth of the matter is that the world hates a martyr. This is the last attitude the martyr wants, since he is so set on the notion that his suffering just has to touch the heartstrings of those close to him. It touches their strings all right, but not in the heart. It's the nerves that get touched, because the martyr is trying to act aggressively even though he denies it. But the person for whom the martyrdom is being acted out senses clearly that he is being attacked. That's precisely why martyrs are not popular any more, and it probably accounts for the reason why they were fed to the lions two thousand years ago. We wouldn't tolerate such inhumane treatment today, but what we do to the martyr today is something almost as unkind. We give in to him. This encourages him to be more self-pitying because he's been rewarded for his tear-jerking performance.

If you don't believe that long-suffering people are disliked for their display of pain, then just look at how easily people pass by beggars. There the poor devils sit, in rain and in sunshine, crippled legs tucked up under half-empty trousered legs, or blind eyes staring into a black sky, and all they want is for you to buy a pencil from them. A coin from every passer-by would give them some of the amenities of life. But have you seen every fifth person even give a beggar a coin? Not very often, I'll bet. And why not? Because we feel so guilty for not being in the shape he is in that we look away. Or we don't give him alms because we think he is using his infirmity to squeeze money out of us. Unfortunately people are turned off by self-pitiers, even where their justification for feeling sorry for themselves is enormous. Imagine how much less pity you will get from your friend or your spouse over the trivial things you want him to pity you for. If people will pass by even though you are blind and lame, how do you expect a positive reaction from them when all you have to complain about is the fact that you haven't been to the cinema for two weeks?

Self-pitiers of the world, stop it! You are using a method of control that works only on the stupid and weak and that makes a first-class fool out of you also. There are better ways of getting what you want out of life—for example, standing up for yourself, not worrying about how many people love you, accepting things as they are if you can't change them, not building up things out of proportion or believing you must have your way at all times and will die if you are frustrated. Make those changes in your life and I guarantee there will be far less self-pity in your life and far less depression as well.

5

OTHER-PITY

We now come to the third and last major reason for psychological depression: other-pity. This has its problems over learning new attitudes, as I will show you. In this instance, however, you will find yourself feeling guilty for *not* taking too seriously the problems that others have.

Just as it is perfectly possible to get depressed and gloomy by pitying yourself, there is no reason whatever that you shouldn't become low-spirited and moody when you pity another person. It makes sense, doesn't it? In fact, if I wanted to really generalize, I could even make out a case for there being only two essential causes for depression: self-blame and pity. Pity applied in any direction can depress you. Pity yourself, pity others, even pity animals or things, such as a city, a landscape, a plane. I remember getting quite gloomy years ago when I had to drive my car to the scrapyard. It had broken down and wasn't worth repairing. To understand my feelings about leaving that car, however, you should know that it was the first car I bought all by myself; I did a great deal of work upholstering it and painting it (even with a shaving brush) and most of all, it had taken me on many long and carefree journeys, now to come to its final grave in a cold and desolate scrapyard. As I walked out of the place, I turned for one last look at my beautiful friend who had been so faithful through so many trying days, and as I saw it among all those ugly wrecks, my heart almost broke. I felt sorry for my car. It didn't deserve such an end, but there wasn't anything I could do about it. Every once in a while I wonder what happened to my little car and what it looks like today.

So getting depressed about a lovely city dying, your birthplace changing over the years, or your dog being run over, is all too natural a reaction and comes under the heading of other-pity.

The Fear of Being Callous

One of the biggest reasons other-pity is so common is the guilt that people feel for *not* being depressed over the misfortune of others. Not being depressed at a funeral could be understood as being rude and callous. Not getting miserable strikes others as being indifferent and uncaring. So people will give out emotions not just because they really do feel upset but because they think they *should* show emotions if an unhappy event occurs. Social etiquette practically demands that certain events be accompanied by very specific emotions. A mouse in a room full of people has got to get the women screaming. It wouldn't be normal if they didn't scream, even if there was no way in the world for the mouse to get up the lady's leg. If they all wore slacks and their trouser legs were tucked into ski socks, the women wouldn't think of not screaming. The situation simply demands this stereotyped behaviour.

It is particularly difficult not to respond to situations where compassion is expected. To be calm about pain or personal loss is often viewed as cruel and uncaring. It need be neither, but to show calmness and lack of intense emotion simply gives people the impression we don't care about the person's plight.

What would you think of someone who helped his friend into an ambulance because of a broken leg but then immediately returned to the football game? Sounds hard, doesn't it? Yet, if the man saw to it that everything possible was done for his friend, if he was sure that the friend's parents were notified and that they would be receiving their son at the hospital, then wouldn't it seem reasonable that he had done all he could and might he not just as well return to his game and have fun? I suppose that still strikes you as unfeeling, but only because you have been taught to think of caring for others always in terms of how upset you get. People find it difficult to believe that undemonstrative people can truly feel intensely or that well-adjusted people can put tragedy out of their minds without treating the tragedy as a trifle.

The Irrational Ideas That Cause Other-pity

Depending on how you look at it, there are one or two irrational ideas that create other-pity. The first is that unhappiness is externally caused, that we are made disturbed by others, and that our emotions have nothing to do with the way we view things. The second is that one should be upset and disturbed over other people's problems and disturbances.

Unhappiness is not externally caused, but frustrations frequently are. What happens to our frustrations usually depends upon us—whether or not we will be disturbed. If we vigorously challenge the idea that frustrations at point A need to upset us at point C, we will eventually get to the point where we will be able to think our way out of feeling wretched over another person's miseries. Practically any experience can be accepted with serenity if one works at thinking rationally about it. People have faced the firing squad, terminal cancer, starvation, all without having a psychotic depression.

So, the next time you see a starving infant on your TV screen remember that what you saw was most regrettable but not capable of disturbing you unless you let it. And if you see a live starved infant, you needn't get depressed either, unless you allow yourself to. Instead of having a nervous breakdown over the starving infant, wrap him up in a blanket, give him some food, and get him to a hospital post haste.

The second idea behind other-pity is simply that you think you ought to get upset because others are upset or are in trouble. Now why in heaven's name *should* you be? Does your suffering help the victim? Are you more able to be of assistance because you have gone and upset yourself mightily over his problems? If so, how? Do you mean to tell me that you wouldn't know how to help someone unless you first worked yourself up into a lather? If so, then why are we being told all the time to keep cool, not to lose our heads, and that easy does it? But no, we still usually get excited, flustered, and depressed first, and then, after we have had a minor emotional fit, decide we had better do something. Isn't that a waste of time and energy? How much better our performance would be if we could really size up a predicament quickly, keep our cool, and swing into action even though we are dealing with a tragedy, and thereby truly be of efficient assistance.

This is not too often the sequence unless the person has had considerable experience of tragedy. Rescue workers, doctors in the Armed Forces, physicians—all these are people trained in dealing with human beings in great distress without falling apart. In fact, we count on their keeping their wits about them and we wouldn't have anything to do with them if they couldn't separate the other party's suffering from their own. In their training they are watched for this trait, the ability to have compassion without excessive sympathy, to show concern without being over-concerned. If they cannot demonstrate this, they will not get far in their training. This ability to stand apart from suffering would be impossible unless these professionals actually agreed with the idea that unhappiness is not externally caused, and that they do not have to get depressed or upset because the people they are helping are depressed or upset.

Concern versus Over-concern

Any civilized person feels for the sufferings of his fellow man. The man who does not have empathy or sensitivity for what people go through is obviously half-witted, moronic, or a write-off. Caring for the plight of one's fellow man is the hallmark of civilized man. But caring too much is not. That is the important line you must draw if you want to stay healthy.

'How do I know when I'm caring too much instead of just caring?' you may ask. Simple. When you hurt. When you start getting depressed and gloomy or angry, that's when you are caring too much for the other person and that's when you are acting irrationally. Yes, irrationally, because your hurt is only adding misery to his misery. What your friend wanted from you was not for you to be pained and depressed. He expected you to pull *him* up to your level of cheerfulness, not let him pull you down to his level of despair.

A perfect example of how other-pity seems perfectly noble but was really very harmful and ineffectual was the case of a social worker who saw me about her depressions. I quickly determined that she couldn't take the sorrow she saw every day as she went on her rounds of the ghetto. After returning home to her comfortable flat in the evening, she would think about all the misery she had seen that day, and the weight of other people's burdens became so great she couldn't eat. Eventually she became more and more listless, until on some days she couldn't even return to her work. Our conversation was something like this.

'Mrs Angelo, you've got to stop caring so much for those people you want to help or you won't get over this depression. The thing that's really depressing you is your belief that you *should* be upset and disturbed over other people's problems and disturbances.'

'Yes, that's it exactly. I do think I should be upset for those poor children, those dirty rooms where there's no sunshine, and where the adults can only sit around all day and go crazy. It breaks my heart to see that day after day.'

'*It* does not break your heart, Mrs Angelo. *You* break it. You keep telling yourself that you *should* be disturbed, that their problems have *got* to upset you, and that you have no control of your emotions in this situation whatever. If you would think those daft ideas over very carefully and stop believing you had to be upset over others' problems, I assure you your blues would lift overnight.'

'But how am I supposed just to push those memories out of my mind? I see misery day in and day out. I just can't go home and forget it,' was her protesting reply.

'I'm glad to hear you can't forget what you see during the day, for otherwise you'd be very callous and I'd suggest you needed treatment to give you a sense of human feeling for your fellow men. But honestly, Mrs Angelo, do you have to care so much that you get disturbed? If you really believed you didn't need to be upset, would you be?'

'No, I suppose not. But how can I possibly convince myself I can look at that poor human condition every day and not get depressed?'

'By thinking through your irrational ideas very

thoroughly and asking yourself if they make sense. First, you know from what I've told you before that *you* upset *yourself*; things can't. Secondly, since you're so cut up because of all the misery you see in the world, what can you do to relieve it? Have you dug in and cleaned up a whole house? Have you been down to the Town Hall and raised a rumpus? Have you even written a letter to your M.P., or a letter to your local newspaper?'

'No, I am sorry to say I haven't. But I see your point. Instead of getting depressed, I should get angry.'

'I prefer the word 'indignant'. You should protest, fight, raise your voice, get some action going. That might change conditions in the slums. But instead, being the sweet person you are who gets all bent out of shape because of the poverty she sees all day, you go home and add to the misery you're complaining about. How clever is that and how much do those people who need your help appreciate that? You feel so much for their prob-lems that you get ill and can't get back to work the next day to help them. What good is that?'

Fortunately, Mrs Angelo could quickly see how foolish and unnecessary her behaviour and symptoms were. She stuck out her chin, stopped being an emotional dishmop and seldom missed a day's work thereafter.

Another example of how wasteful and even dangerous other-pity is came to me through a kindly old gentleman, a Mr Wall. He read a great deal and knew a lot about politics. The thing that infuriated him was crooked politics and how it took advantage of the little business-man. His brother was ruined by petty local politics, and this hurt Mr Wall so much that he became restless, couldn't sleep, and got very embittered. The worst part of it was the fact that he had a very bad heart and it didn't do him any good at all to get worked up over

the millions of injustices in this world. But Mr Wall
identified so closely with the underdogs and felt so
deeply for the hurt they experienced in this unfair world
that he almost burst even while he was telling me about
it. He got red in the face, his breath was laboured, and
he perspired as he told me about injustice and suffering
in the world. It frightened me as he went on, because I
could see him have a cardiac arrest there in the office.
Finally, to quieten him down I screamed over his voice
and reassured him that I too knew the world was a
stinking place but that we both had better get used to the
smell. I praised him for his concern for his fellow men
but also pointed out that his having a heart attack and
bleeding psychologically was not the solution his dis-
advantaged friends were hoping for. What had he done
about crooked politics? Had he run for political office
himself, or helped someone campaign, or stuffed en-
velopes at an election headquarters?

He had done none of these, so we debated for a
while about the utter stupidity of his nearly killing himself over conditions he did nothing to relieve aside from
shouting and complaining. Eventually he learned to
accept ugly reality more gracefully, although at his age
and in his condition he could not actively correct or
contribute to the causes he honoured. The depression and
the agitation lifted nicely and when I last heard from
him he was still alive. I hope he didn't get himself worked
up too much over the problems and disturbances of
others and die of a heart attack.

In both of these examples, it's easy to see how a
healthy and kindly concern for the welfare of others
was converted unwittingly into marked depression in
one case, and almost death in the other. Over-concern,
not concern, was the culprit. Each of these fine individuals could easily have detected when they began caring

too much: the moment they realized they were upset they could also have realized they were being irrational and self-defeating.

Emotional Blackmail

One of the most serious consequences of pitying others is the malicious use to which that human weakness can be put. For instance, if I know you have the tendency to feel excessive sympathy for me, that puts me in a position of control should I want to use it. Just imagine what I can get away with. I can make you invite me to your home, I can make you marry whomever I choose, and I can make you work in whatever occupation I think best. How much more control does anyone need? If I can do all that, then I have your soul also. Does this sound far fetched? Then listen to this: I can't tell you how many people have told me that they married their spouses because he or she threatened suicide. How many parents have forced their children to live at home far into adulthood just so that they wouldn't be alone? Haven't you ever been manipulated because someone used your own guilt feelings to make you give in to him? Practically everybody has used this technique and has had it used upon himself. It often works beautifully simply because you have the complete co-operation of the person you want to control.

Don't let the suffering of others turn you away from what you consider your best interests. If you feel strongly about marrying Roger and your father goes into a depression over the prospect, don't give up your fiancé to please your father or you will be accepting his emotional blackmail.

There are several terribly important facts to remember if you want to avoid being emotionally blackmailed.

First, no matter how upset the other person gets over your behaviour or your plans, do not blame yourself for his state of mind. Your father, or whoever is blackmailing you, is upsetting himself. Tell him so.

Secondly, when the blackmailer tries to tell you he is doing all this for love of you, don't believe him. The blackmailer hasn't any real desire to let you be an independent human being at all. He will be happy only when he gets his way. So he's hoping to make you so uncomfortable with his tears, moaning, and anxiety that you will take pity on his poor soul and give him his way. He is really interested almost exclusively in his own end, not in yours.

Thirdly, don't let someone's threat of suicide get you down. If he uses that weapon on you, tell him instantly that you refuse to be responsible for his death, that he has control over his life, that the whole idea is a rotten trick, and that if it makes him happy to die, then do. This is not as callous as it sounds. To do otherwise is perhaps to induce the person to try suicide in the hope of getting you to give in. But if you make it crystal clear that you regret his taking such an action while at the same time you grant him the freedom to do it, you may be amazed at how this nonsense stops. Only recently I heard of another case of a daughter whose father threatened to kill himself numerous times in order to manipulate his family. One fine day the daughter answered the phone. Good old dad made the same threat, but this time daughter took a deep sigh and candidly told her father that if that is what he really wanted to do, to go ahead. He never threatened his family again.

Fourthly, pitying others weakens them. Instead of bolstering up their courage, as you think you are doing, your sentimentality is merely telling them how hopeless you think they are and how you fully understand why they should be depressed. The individual already is telling himself: 'Poor me. I'm too inadequate to deal with this issue.' And you come along with your other-pity and in effect say to him, 'Poor you, you really are too inadequate to handle this issue.' How in the world is the self-pitier supposed to get stronger through that treatment? Obviously he can't.

One young boy who was brought to me because of his excessive timidity was the unwitting victim of his mother's great affection for him. He was one of the most protected children I had ever seen. His well-meaning mother wouldn't allow him a bicycle when all the other boys were learning to ride, because Mike was supposedly 'too unco-ordinated'. By the same token Mike didn't attempt swimming, roller skating, or football until his classmates were quite accomplished at these sports.

At first Mike protested, but his mother worried so much over him that the poor chap began to soak up her pity for him to the point where he lost his natural youthful adventurousness and spontaneity. Instead, Mike wouldn't risk a thing if it could conceivably hurt him.

Happily his mother was really a caring and intelligent person and could follow my reasoning quickly. I instructed her to stop the pity and to let the boy take his chances. Instead of her turning the colour of a white sheet when he wanted to go swimming with his mates, I ordered her to control her anxiety for her son's sake, put on a brave and cheerful smile, and send him off with a pat on the rump. Yes, he might drown, I agreed, but what was happening to him anyway? Wasn't he slowly dying of boredom and excessive safety? Life is a gamble and there's nothing you or I can do about removing all its dangers. Mike's mother had tried to spare her son some of those hardships and dangers, but in reality she had placed him in the greatest danger of all: not being able to face new situations, not developing the proper skills to enable him to avoid danger, not developing in him a sense of self-assurance which is far better than a lonely corner. Certainly, he might get his shins skinned or his leg broken, but so what? A broken leg will heal easily in about four to six weeks, but a broken spirit may take a lifetime to mend.

Mike's mother did her homework well. She didn't give the usual clues to him which always signalled her concern, and this gave him new courage. She didn't twist her handkerchief, bite her lip, shed tears, stiffen with anxiety, or ask a lot of questions implying that he was walking into death's jaws every time he wanted to cross two streets to go to a sweet shop.

At first the mother simply forced herself to let her son go and it nearly made a depressive out of her. For a time I thought I was going to have to treat her for *her* emotional problem. As Mike became more and more of a normal boy, however, and as he became slightly aggressive and occasionally acted like a tearaway, she relaxed as she saw his new strength. He learned to ride better, to swim as well as the next boy, and to play a decent game of football. The few minor injuries he suffered were fortunately not so bad as to make her go back on her new approach. Luck frequently plays a bigger role in our emotional lives and in our whole development than we realize.

Other-pity Can Frequently Cause Legal Injustice

Justice often calls for stiff measures. Being soft when you should be firm can cause all sorts of unfairness. And what causes more sloppy sentimentality than other-pity?

Nothing! Getting gushy and soft about another person can cause you to misunderstand him cómpletely and to treat him in ways not really in his own best interests.

Take the case of Mr Polin. He drank too much, always drove when he drank, and had clocked up a list of accidents while under the influence of alcohol. None of this seriously interfered with his drinking, however, because he simply continued to be careless about his behaviour and not to realize the danger in which he placed others. One night he narrowly missed hitting a pedestrian, but he did smash up a parked car.

Among the jurors was one of my patients, a Mrs Clark, whose major psychological problem was other-pity. I had worked with her on this problem for several months and she was in excellent control of this tendency when she was asked to sit on the jury.

On the day the jury retired, Mrs Clark had a most interesting experience. She found herself completely alone in wanting to find Mr Polin guilty as charged and deserving a heavy fine plus a short jail sentence. She had no pity for the defendant and believed a good spanking might make him grow up and act responsibly. The rest of the jury, however, wanted to soft-pedal Mr Polin's accident and let him off very easy in view of the little damage actually caused to the car in question. This did not satisfy my patient, because she was far more concerned about the need to make a solid impression on Mr Polin than about the need to judge him solely on this one incident.

She said: 'It occurred to me that the entire jury was suffering from other-pity just as I had done all my life. I knew the signs well and could just see the wheels going around in their heads. They were probably telling themselves that he was a nice bloke and didn't mean to run into that car; that he would surely learn by this experience

despite the fact that he had done this sort of thing before; and that they'd feel badly if they caused him to lose
money or spend time in jail. Well, as you know, I've
been there and I know how feeling sorry for someone
else can really mess you up, even to the point where
you're being hurt by not learning the right lessons.

'The whole jury were surprised and shocked at my
insistence that we make this man see his behaviour for
what it was. They wanted me to give in to them, but I
wouldn't. And do you know, after several hours of
debating the case I had won them all over to my side.
And best of all, I believe they felt pleased with their
decision, because they could focus on the good they
were eventually doing him rather than the immediate
relief he would have got. They overcame their other-
pity and could deal with this problem quite easily, just
as I did.'

Mrs Clark had good reason to speak so knowingly.
Part of her difficulty as a mother was her inability to be
firm with her children because of the temporary frustration her restrictions would cause them. So, instead of
insisting they study, she let them go out and play in the
evenings. Instead of making sure that they practised their
instruments, she let their early musical interests wane
and disappear. Instead of making them clean up their
rooms and help around the house, she did the work
herself. She pitied them whenever she expected work or
responsibility from them. They sensed that she was an
easy touch for a long face, so they put on the 'poor me'
act and got her to back down on practically every one
of her rules. In the end they wound up spoiled and un-
manageable brats whom she had trouble liking.

This was a serious injustice to her children. Her pity
for them made her weak and stupid. They ran the house
and messed up their lives as a result. When she went into

court, she could sense how this drama was being re-enacted, but this time she was prepared to give a mature, firm reaction rather than a whimpering, pitying reaction, and she was prepared to do that man a service by being tough on him even if she had to take an unpopular stand with the rest of the jury.

An immense amount of injustice is committed in the name of love. It is time to redefine the word 'love' and expand it into something that includes the idea of caring for someone beyond the immediate moment, for what is satisfying now is often bad for us in the near future. Other-pity only considers the current frustration, not the frustrations that lie months and years ahead.

Other-pitiers Produce Self-pitiers

Of all the faults with other-pity, none is so damaging as the creation of self-pitiers. To see this, all you have to do is watch a mother and a child in a park. The child falls and hurts himself, but he tries to bear up against the pain. His mother has not seen what happened because she's reading a book. Her son then comes up to her, a pained expression on his face, holding his kneecap where it was skinned. At the moment of realization her heart melts for her little boy, she cuddles him in her arms, holds him tight, makes a catastrophe of the skinned knee, and signals to him that he ought to cry because he has to be in awful pain. And that is precisely what the child then does: he pities himself and *then* breaks into howling sobs. When this scene is enacted often enough, the end result has to be one thing and one thing only: a self-pitier of the first order.

If the mother would curb her maternal enthusiasm, recognize her son's accident, even tell him that it must hurt and that he is free to cry if he wants to, and then wash the wound off with her handkerchief, she will have shown him an entirely different way of responding to such mishaps. She will have been caring and compassionate without being gushing and pitying. Nothing in this last description could hurt her son. It could only help him. But there is a great deal in the former method that might stunt his growth.

The simple truth of the matter is that self-pity comes easily enough to human beings, but when it's backed with maternal or paternal love, watch out! Once a family of children get the 'poor you' treatment for a few years, they soak up that nonsense so thoroughly that they can't think of others any longer, only of themselves.

One of the sorriest cases of other-pity backfiring which I have ever encountered was that of Mrs Bee. She was one of those good mothers, always sacrificing for her children and husband, going without so that they could have, and being glad of the opportunity to serve. All her feelings were so completely invested in her family they truly began to believe that the world revolved around them, that mother was there to serve them, and that they had a positive right to be highly indignant if they didn't get their self-indulgent ways. So her husband began to go out with the boys because he enjoyed it. When she kindly asked to be taken along sometimes or to be taken out at the weekend he felt so put upon that she felt guilty for asking.

Though she worked for pin money for a few extra-nice clothes for herself, she always wound up getting something new for her whining daughters who thought that their mother owed them a new wardrobe every season. After a while they helped less and less with the housework, and even her asking for her husband's help to make the girls behave didn't have the desired effect. When she reached the point where she could clearly see she had become a maid and personal servant she still couldn't express her wrath but instead pitied herself and phoned me about her thoughts of suicide.

My advice to her was clear and simple. 'Stop feeling so much for that crew of yours. Make them toe the line. Stand up to them. Let them scream like stuck pigs if they want to, but don't give in on any pretext.'

Alas, the advice was simple enough but impossible for this well-trained martyr to follow. All it took was one firm, 'No!' from her husband, and an indignant exit from the room by her daughters and she was a defeated creature once more. She didn't see me again, but I can clearly guess that the pattern at home is the same and that she will continue to be depressed from other-pity and self-pity.

'If It Hadn't Been for You'

A very common way others seduce you into feeling sorry for them is to place the blame for their disturbances on you. Then you are supposed to see how awful you have been and do an about-face by giving your accuser everything he wants.

A young wife came to me once, very much depressed because of the great guilt she felt over frequently upsetting her husband, and over the remorse she felt for him as a result of her mistakes. This at first sounded as though she had a good deal of insight into her marriage, but in order to be sure I questioned her.

'Mrs Schafer, can you give me an example of what you are referring to?'

'Certainly,' was her reply. 'Last week the police came to my house asking for my husband. They had a warrant for his arrest for car theft. They claimed the car my husband bought last week was really stolen. I was shocked, of course, and simply couldn't believe it. But it was true, all right. He told me he had bought it and he made up a lie about how much it had cost and how he had financed it, and if I didn't believe him, I could go to the bank and see a withdrawal last week for the amount of the down payment. When the police and I both put him on the spot, he insisted he'd stolen it because I made him do it.'

'You made him steal a car?' I asked.

'That's what he insisted. It seems I expressed a desire for a new car recently and then he insisted that if it hadn't been for me asking for a new car, he wouldn't have been compelled to go out and steal one. He says I'm always making him do things he doesn't want to do. And I suppose he's right. After all, if I didn't make the requests in the first place, he wouldn't have any reason to steal things for me when he can't afford them. When he put it this way I felt so guilty for being so selfish and inconsiderate, and I felt so sorry for the burdens and pressures I put on my husband.'

It was quite apparent from her strange tale that her husband was a sly old fox. I used to marvel when I heard such ridiculous accounts, but I don't any more. Now I'm nearly sick at the utter gullibility of some people. Can anyone actually believe that she *meant* every word she told me? She did indeed!

I was able to help her wake up by showing her first of all that she cannot make someone steal anything unless she puts a gun to his head and threatens to blow his brains out unless he steals. And even then she can't make him do it if he really doesn't want to, because he can always decide to die rather than live under those conditions. Secondly, I pointed out that her husband was a spineless wonder or he would have had the nerve to tell her he didn't have the money for a car. He could

have told himself that having his wife think poorly of
him would have been unpleasant but hardly catastrophic.
Had he done so he could easily have allowed her innocent
comment to go in one ear and out the other.

The sly old fox didn't do that, however, because he had
too much abnormal pride to admit he wasn't a magician
or a millionaire. In view of these faults which he clearly
possessed it was easy to pose the logical question, 'Now,
Mrs Schafer, how can you blame yourself for actions for
which your husband was clearly responsible?'

'I think I can follow you so far, but what about his
argument that none of that would have happened if I
hadn't expressed a desire for a new car? You must admit
that all of this probably wouldn't have happened if I
hadn't made the request in the first place. Isn't that so?'

'Yes,' I agreed. 'Perhaps none of this would have
happened if you hadn't made the suggestion to have a
new car. However, just because you did make the
suggestion doesn't mean you're responsible for what
followed. You have an indirect share of the responsibility,
I agree, because you did make the request. But if that's
true, then there are a whole host of people who should
also share in the guilt for this act and feel sorry for what
they're doing to your poor husband.'

'Like whom?'

'Like the car manufacturer for making such lovely
cars. And like the company he works for because they
don't pay him enough to buy expensive cars when he
wants them. And like the social system we live in that
says we must pay for things we want. Aren't all these
parties also indirectly guilty for your husband's act?
But would you seriously hold them responsible and say
they made him steal?'

The debate went on for the remainder of our talk
together, but as we drew to a close she could begin to

see my reasoning and see her husband's antics for what they were. After a time she could see him as a weak fellow, very eager to have his wife's love and foolish enough to do almost anything to assure himself of her respect, but also as someone who was too defensive to see his own behaviour clearly and who then played on the sympathies of others by making them feel guilty over an innocent act while at the same time feeling much sympathy for him.

Learn this lesson early in your life and you will be spared a great deal of grief: no one can make you do anything unless by force. People do what they do because they want to or because they are afraid to turn you down because they want your approval so badly. Either way, that is something they are responsible for. So never let them blame you or make you feel sorry for them when they have voluntarily committed a folly.

A Few Final Tips

1. Your depression will end even if you do nothing about it. So don't despair when you get low. Sunshine is just over the horizon! That is one of the few fortunate features about depression which we cannot report about anger, for instance, or about fear. It is possible to be timid, fearful, shy, and anxious for practically the whole of one's life. And it is perfectly possible to be resentful, bitter, hateful, or angry for practically every day of one's life. But when you have an episode of depression you can count on one thing for certain: whether you take medicine for it or not, it will end; and if you do nothing about it, the depression will end.

No matter how wretched and gloomy you may feel at times, try to remember that this feeling of despair will one day be past history. You can be absolutely sure about that. You don't have to kill yourself to get over your misery, all you need is patience!

2. The ideas and suggestions I've put down in this book are sound and will help anyone suffering from psychological depression. I personally have had great success in helping some people for whom, before I formulated this theory of depression, I would have had to cross my fingers and hope that I could do them some good. My approach to the problem now has relieved some of the most stubborn depressions I have encountered in my practice.

Further Types of Psychological Treatment Available

Persistent or severe depression may need more radical treatment than the self-help described in this book. Anti-depressant drugs and electro-convulsive therapy will alleviate the symptoms of depression but do not attack the cause. The root of the problem lies in an individual's attitudes and feelings towards himself and others and this can be treated through various methods of psycho-therapy. The following are the most common in Great Britain at the moment.

Psychoanalysis pioneered by Freud (and developed in different directions by Jung, Adler and others) aims at helping people to resolve emotional conflicts which are seen as being rooted in the experiences of early child-hood. Specific techniques of analysis of a person's unconscious mind are used, in regular sessions, (normally five times a week) over a period of years.

Dynamic psychotherapy. Psychotherapy is dynamic wherever it aims at changing or developing the personality by handling unconscious material to resolve conflicts.

Dynamic psychotherapy therefore includes psychoanalytic interpretation, but it also uses other methods of approach of a lesser depth and intensity. Many children and adolescents receive psychotherapy free from trained child psychotherapists at Child Guidance Clinics under the National Health Service or local authorities. Very few adults indeed receive psychoanalysis or dynamic psychotherapy of an intensive kind under the N.H.S. A classical analysis can take up to 750 sessions at about five pounds per session. Moreover there are only about 400 fully trained psychotherapists and the majority of these practise in London outside the National Health Service.

Supportive psychotherapy (a term widely used by psychiatrists) means psychotherapy which aims at assisting people to understand their everyday problems, often in terms of past experience, and to adjust to them so that they become more tolerable, rather than trying to change or develop their personalities. Frequency of interviews varies but may be as little as three or four times a year. Supportive psychotherapy is used in the many cases where a person is unwilling or unable to make the kind of fundamental change aimed at in dynamic psychotherapy.

Casework is the name given to a social worker's dealings with a person's personal problems over a fairly long period. It is often the equivalent of supportive psychotherapy but may have more dynamic elements.

Counselling like supportive psychotherapy and casework, is an attempt to explore a person's problems with him and to promote a helpful adjustment to any basic problems which may exist. Counselling may be undertaken by members of other professions, such as teachers or ministers of religion, or by people specializing in a particular type of problem, e.g. marriage guidance or student counselling.

Behaviour therapy is based on the principal that people learn neurotic patterns of behaviour and that they can also be taught to learn normal patterns of behaviour. By administering a small electric shock every time a particular fear is experienced, anxious and fearful people overcome their worries. Alternatively, the therapist may relax or hypnotize the patient and then ask him to imagine the things he fears until he gradually loses his fear of them.

Group therapy While treatments have traditionally been developed on a one to one basis there is an increasing movement towards group therapy. In this treatment discussions take place regularly between a group of people in the presence of a psychotherapist who tries to help them understand their problems and interaction. Group therapy tends to be dynamic in its effects and may not be suited to everyone.

Further Reading

Casson, F.R.C., *Anxiety, Nervousness and Depression.* British Medical Association 1971.

Kenny, Bill and Whitehead, Tony, *Insight — A Guide to Psychiatry and Psychiatric Service.* Croom Helm 1973.

Mitchell, A.R.K., *Psychological Medicine in General Practice.* Balliere 1971.

Mitchell, A.R.K., *Shades of Grey.* MIND, National Association for Mental Health 1974.

Rycroft, Charles, *Anxiety and Neurosis.* Pelican 1970.

Watts, C.A.H., *Depression — The Blue Plague.* Priory Press 1973.